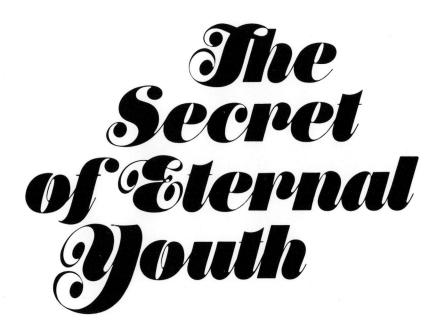

The Secret of Eternal Youth

REJUVENATION THROUGH DR. NIEHANS' CELL THERAPY

PETER M. STEPHAN

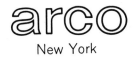

arco
New York

I would like to extend my thanks to Miss Jean Soward for her help with the editorial preparation of this manuscript.

Published by ARCO PUBLISHING COMPANY, INC.
219 Park Avenue South, New York, N.Y. 10003

This book is being published simultaneously in
Great Britain under the title *Cell Therapy*.

Second Printing, 1972

Library of Congress Catalog Number 71-158467
ISBN 0-668-02489-5

Printed in the United States of America

Contents

*cells in body repair . . . degeneration and loss of
reproductive power . . . refutation of popular fallacies
. . . revitalization not rejuvenation . . . Abderhalden
resistance-ferment reaction test . . . length of
treatment . . . infectious diseases.*

Contents

Introduction

EVERYONE is interested in health, if not consciously, for its own sake, then indirectly as a means of getting the best and most out of life. Similarly, everyone is secretly haunted by the fear of old age, decrepit, unwholesome old age. The fact of increasing age has inevitably to be accepted; but need there be any inevitablity about the disagreeable accompaniments?

Most of us have had the experience, at some time or other, of meeting an ailing friend or acquaintance who exclaimed wistfully: "If only I could have a new stomach" (or a few new arteries, or other pieces of vital internal mechanism), "I'd be all right." The speaker tosses off the words with the sort of courageous light-heartedness which gains him sympathy, of course, but also pity, for it is tacitly assumed on both sides that without major and, since it is still experimental, dangerous spare-part surgery, there is little possibility of this piece of wishful thinking being transformed into fact.

That assumption is no longer valid. Biological running repairs, leading to renewals and replacements within the human organism, are an accomplished fact of current medical practice, even if as yet carried out by only a handful of pioneering practitioners. This repair process—accomplished without drugs and without surgery—is not quite so simple as putting a new part into a car engine or watch, but, in terms of restoration of working order and increased efficiency, the results are entirely comparable. The seeming miracles this process can accomplish are the logical consequences of ever-deepening insights into the complexities of the structure, the growth patterns and, above all, the chemistry of living tissue in healthy and in pathological states. They represent a new therapeutic technique of co-operation with natural forces by exploiting biological processes to the extent of "fooling" Nature herself, and thus giving her a helping hand in need.

Professor Niehans himself is an astonishingly young octogenarian, with vitality and working capacity not often found in men half his age. His own zest and youthfulness demonstrate the sincerity of his promise that cell injections "put more life into one's years, and more years into one's life."

This technique is the Niehans' method of cell therapy, often called popularly "Niehans' Youth Injections." Although this is in fact a true description, it is also one which, unless backed by impartial and objective information about the process involved, can produce understandable feelings of scepticism. Where such scepticism exists it stems from the fact that so far what little information the public has been able to glean about cell therapy has come from highly-colored and, for the most part, grossly exag-

[8]

gerated newspaper reports, favorable and the reverse, which have tended either to paint a rosy picture of a universal panacea, wonder cure and rejuvenator, or to sound a warning against possible imposition by skilled quackery.

To correct such erroneous impressions is partly the purpose of this book.

Its other and more important purpose is to give as much detailed information about cell therapy and its derivatives as there is available, thus enabling people alert and intelligent enough to seek scientific information for themselves to understand its basic principles and also perhaps to answer for themselves the question: Could this therapy do something for me?

1

Patients

CELL THERAPY is a subject which is still to some extent cloaked in mystery. While it could be called the "in" people's treatment, from the general public's point of view it is still in its infancy.

This is largely because after treatment most patients are reluctant to admit the source of their new-found health, vitality and improved appearance. They seem to prefer to keep the whole thing dark and pretend that it just happened. "All my own work," they infer as they accept the compliments of friends and relations on their attractive new personality and looks.

But despite the apparent conspiracy of silence, so many celebrities have resorted to the treatment made famous by the controversial Swiss doctor, Professor Paul Niehans, that, whatever efforts they may have made to hide the fact, news of it has leaked out. The list of the eminent who are either known to have had cell therapy, or reliably reputed to have had it, runs into hundreds, even thousands of names: from the Duke and Duchess of Windsor to the late General Eisenhower during his presidency; from King Ibn Saud and other Middle East potentates to Gloria Swanson and Marlene Dietrich, who makes little secret of her repeat injections every five years.

Ram Gopal, the Hindu dancer, has had cell therapy; so have actor Bob Cummings, artist Georges Braque, Furt-wängler, the conductor. General de Gaulle is said to have had injections. Charlie Chaplin, too, and the Duke of Sutherland who, far from trying to hide the fact, seems rather proud of it. Even Noel Coward, after claiming for years that he was "too fearful for such things," finally admitted to a "rejuvenating shot" during a television interview about twelve months ago.

It was Pope Pius XII, then head of the Roman Catholic Church, who first brought the name of Niehans and knowledge of his work to the attention of the general public.

Early in 1954 Niehans was summoned to the Pontiff's bedside, having been recommended by Sister Pasqualina, his Bavarian nurse, and by the head of the Papal Swiss Guard. No treatment was given on that occasion, but some months later the Pope's condition again gave cause for alarm and it was officially announced that a Swiss specialist had been called in.

The specialist was Niehans, on his second visit, this time to Castel Gandolfo, where cell treatment *was* carried out. It was the eleventh hour in every respect. Pius XII was seventy-eight, emaciated, racked by gastric pain and daily failing in strength. Niehans stayed three weeks to supervise his patient's reaction to injection. He had the satisfaction of observing that the incessant hiccups, which

[12]

had been one of the Pope's most distressing symptoms, had completely vanished; also, for one in his condition, the patient was eating and sleeping well again.

Before he left Castel Gandolfo that summer Doctor Niehans and his English wife, Coralis, were photographed with his distinguished patient restored to health. The framed photograph now stands in the drawing room of the doctor's home high above the lake of Geneva about a mile from his clinic at Burier-Vevey, near Montreux. In the same room are a pair of gold cuff-links embossed with the keys of St. Peter—the Pope's personal gift.

A chance misfortune brought Niehans again to the Pope's bedside the following November. Pope Pius XII, always energetic and hard-working, thought nothing of doing things with his own hands if other help were not available when he wanted these things done. On this occasion he had tried to lift a heavy box. The Pope recovered and astonished the world by working at high pressure up to a few days before his death in October 1958, at the age of eighty-two.

In 1955, in recognition of his Swiss doctor's services, Pius XII had appointed Niehans to the chair left vacant in the Pontifical Academy of Sciences by the death of Sir Alexander Fleming, discoverer of penicillin. And in 1956 the Pope publicly endorsed cell therapy before an international gathering of medical men in Rome. Further recognition came in 1958 when Niehans was appointed to a Professorship at the University of Tübingen.

King George VI had just missed becoming a patient in January 1952. By the time Niehans was called, the King lay dying of cancer, after making a shaky recovery from a lung operation. When the King's physicians learned from Niehans that there was nothing he could do they expressed surprise. "But you helped Churchill," they said.

Niehans pointed out that Churchill had been helped while he was still capable of benefiting from help. "I can regenerate an old body," he told them; "can prevent the body from aging before its time, revitalize glands and reduce cholesterol; but there are limits to what I can do."

And it is a fact that Sir Winston Churchill was claimed to be one of those who owed their health and vigor as octogenarians to cell therapy. Novelist Somerset Maugham never made a secret of his treatments. Each time he had a fresh set of injections he gave Press interviews, describing his reactions and declaring that, perhaps after all, he had been a little premature in announcing years ago that he had written his last book.

Konrad Adenauer was also one of the veterans whose physical and mental stamina were attributed to timely biological repair, although he himself refused to discuss the subject. It is known, however, that Niehans paid several visits to the sprightly German Chancellor in the early 1950's, and what Niehans began others could easily carry on, since cell therapy is accepted practice in the highest medical circles in Germany. This practice, unfortunately, is not echoed in Britain. And some of the blame for *unin*-formed public opinion about the exact nature of cell therapy and its effects must be laid at the door of the medical establishment.

Blame for *mis*-informed public opinion—the reason for the often furtive half-ashamed secrecy of the way in which people set about getting their biological repairs done—can

be laid at another door: that of the more sensational organs of the popular Press.

Almost the only information published has been grossly
exaggerated reports of marvelous rejuvenation, restored
physical beauty, sex appeal and attractiveness resulting
in romance at unlikely ages and the mending of broken
marriages.

Even members of the medical profession, while themselves under no illusion about the truth of such stories,
have been influenced by them. Many medical practitioners
in Britain have had cell treatment personally, but always
in conditions of sworn secrecy and surrounded by every
possible security precaution.

Not surprisingly, these fantastic rejuvenation stories
arouse considerable interest in the minds of middle-aged
and elderly women readers of newspapers and magazines.
They come to the consulting room with a vague notion
that they will be given one injection of some miraculous
substance, the patented secret of "this Professor Niehans"
which is both a universal remedy for all ills and a magic
formula for the restoration of youth. They expect to wake
up the morning after receiving it feeling and looking at
least twenty years younger.

They are then rather taken aback by the necessity for a
searching medical examination and other preliminaries
which precede treatment. And disappointed when it has to
be tactfully explained that what they hope for is impossible, a cure against the laws of Nature, something beyond
the reach of science.

For example, it is perhaps unfortunate, but a fact, that
the woman who is about fifty years old and looks her
age, *but who in every other respect is healthy,* cannot ex-

pect any conspicuous result from undergoing cell therapy. If such a patient is quite simply after a spectacular facial rejuvenation she has to be politely but firmly discouraged.

Actually, of course, this hypothetical person of fifty who enjoys perfect health is something of a dodo. In these days when practically everybody suffers from some degree of stress and its neurological, functional and organic consequences, it is very difficult indeed to find the completely healthy middle-aged person.

Due to wear and tear and the increasing stresses of "civilized" life, examination nearly always reveals some degree of premature aging, some pathological changes, some degeneration in the organic, nervous or glandular system. In fact, approximately 80 percent of modern diseases and illnesses are agreed by the medical profession to be "stress conditions," the results of prolonged physical and nervous strain and mental stress.

The middle-aged patient may be primarily concerned with appearance and the obvious signs of lost youth but, in fact, she (or he) proves to be far from healthy: worn, worried, nervous, fidgety and unable to relax, full of fears and anxiety.

Cell therapy is of considerable value in such cases: and in helping to repair the whole human machine it certainly does make the patient feel and look younger.

The sharp lines of stress and strain, the sallow skin, sagging contours and bloodshot eyes of impaired circulation, the pouches under the eyes resulting from lymphatic obstruction, all these depressing signs of an ill-functioning prematurely aged system can be smoothed out in the process of recovery, and often vanish completely.

Overweight or underweight can be corrected; and with

[16]

help from the patient through attention to diet, posture and exercise, the figure itself can be improved in time.

In so far as better health and normalized organic and glandular functioning give these exterior results, the biological repair process set in motion by cell therapy does produce a certain degree of rejuvenation. But it is a comparative, or apparent, rejuvenation. What actually happens is that people so treated are made to look the way Nature intended them to look at their age instead of ten or twenty years older. So, as stressed earlier, it is only the patient who is obsessed with the idea of a marked facial improvement who must be warned, even when her case is otherwise suitable, not to expect the impossible.

The largest group of patients, after the youth and beauty seekers, fall into two categories: those who have worked too hard, and those who have played too hard.

These two groups, the overworked and the overplayed, include a multitude of types, physical conditions and psychological difficulties. Frequently, of course, the effects of overwork and overplay are observable in the one person.

There is the overworked business executive, politician, professional man, actor, anyone in fact who leads a strenuous life and has no choice but to go on leading it. There comes a time when he suddenly feels worn out, notices that he is slowing down, lacking in energy, slipping mentally and physically, unable, in general, to cope with his work and his life as he could in the past; in short, getting old before his time.

If this kind of patient uses common sense after treatment, cell therapy can usually be of considerable help. It will restore his energy and vitality to the fullest extent possible within the laws of Nature.

The man who has played hard all his life, and possibly overworked as well, can be something of a problem. His health is wrecked from burning the candle at both ends for years, and over-indulging in everything—alcohol, sex, drugs. He has contracted all sorts of complaints, especially arteriosclerosis, heart trouble, high blood pressure, cirrhosis of the liver, alcoholism and insomnia, to name but a few.

Cell injections can help to build up a devastated, ruined human system; but in such a case will the rebuilding be any use in the long run? This is the type of patient who tends to disregard warnings and starts all over again the moment his ills are cured. In cases like this the question of where the practitioner's duty and responsibilty lie must also be weighed in the balance.

Another frequent patient is the tired, middle-aged husband suffering from impotence, or decline of the libido. This is generally the result either of sexual over-indulgence in the past, or of prolonged stress in his daily life or of both. It also occurs when the entire libido, all the vital resources of the body, are poured into the patient's work under the spur of some powerful motive like ambition, and he is left with no energy to spare for sex-life.

When impotence in the middle-aged male is due to past over-indulgence, it is accompanied by various other glandular deficiencies and organic disfunctions. These can be restored to normal by cell therapy, but the patient has to be warned that when he has regained his health he must be more economical with his vital powers, and not expect to repeat in middle age the excesses of his youth.

The same warning must apply to the overworked business or professional man suffering from impotence through prolonged stress. If, after a cure, he does not slow down the continuous pressure of his daily work at the old pace he will have just one result: the effects of biological repair in his case will be of short duration.

The middle-aged patient with a history of impotence in his youth belongs to a different category. So does the patient whose impotence is largely psychological and who has taken refuge in drugs, aphrodisiacs and artificial stimulants, or been given hormone treatment in various forms.

Patients in this category are often very reluctant to admit the use of stimulants and sex hormones, and their reticence greatly complicates the treatment of their case.

Prolonged hormone treatment, whether the sex hormones or others, complicates subsequent cell treatment because it inevitably produces a further incapacitation of already underactive glands. Since most glands secrete a variety of hormones, and not just one, the prolonged substitution of a single hormone for the whole series also stops the secretion of the others through the progessive atrophy of the gland.

In the case of the impotent male, the hormone substances may have made his system function temporarily at a better rate and may also have restored libido and sexual potency; but these results will have lasted only so long as the hormone therapy was continued, usually with ever-increasing doses. Sooner or later the patient reaches a state where even the most substantial dose no longer has any effect And this, in many cases, is the moment when he decides to try cell therapy.

Thus it can be seen that if the use of hormones is not admitted, the cell injections may not be suitably composed for the case, and the whole treatment may be a failure.

However, provided the patient at least mentions previous hormone treatments or the use of aphrodisiacs, his cell therapy treatment, which will aim at restoring normal function of affected glands so that at least for a considerable time they produce their own hormones again in natural balanced quantities, can be adjusted and accentuated accordingly.

If the atrophy of the treated glands has not advanced too far, a permanent restoration of normal function is possible. But it is always essential to impress upon the patient the importance of not reverting again to hormone treatment.

Another type of patient who turns up frequently in the cell therapist's consulting room is the so-called hypochondriac. This patient is the despair of his family and of his family doctor—or perhaps doctors—since he is constantly changing his medical adviser in a seemingly hopeless quest for relief from apparently undiagnosable symptoms.

He will have been medically examined again and again, using all the normal methods, including X-rays, blood tests, and so on—always with negative results. The doctor assumes there is nothing physically wrong, a fact which he expresses as tactfully as possible to the patient and more openly to the patient's relatives. With nothing but negative results from exhaustive clinical tests there is only one conclusion: the patient's complaints are non-existent physically; they are psychological and hysterical.

Sometimes this diagnosis is correct. But on the other hand many of these cases do have tangible physical symptoms and real pain. Telling these patients to pull themselves together and stop being a nuisance to themselves and to everyone else does not help. Referring them to a psychiatrist if they are not in fact neurotic is useless.

[20]

It is cases of this kind that Abderhalden Resistance Ferment Reaction Tests, the special tests on which cell therapy is based and which will be explained in detail in later chapters of this book, can come to the rescue and by their minutely accurate diagnosis of conditions which escape all conventional diagnostic methods reveal the truth. In other words, while conventional diagnostic methods reveal only what is pretty far gone, the cell therapy tests catch the small beginnings. The deterioration in one gland or organ would not, of course, cause much trouble. But the total of say twenty or thirty miscellaneous slight dysfunctions can and often does produce the type of patient who is regarded as hysterical.

When this patient has cell treatment to correct the multiple dysfunctions which have been making his or her life a misery, the result is often spectacular and considered a "miracle."

2

Discovery and
Background

FROM the patient's point of view, a shot or two of the right cells is quick and painless; moreover, it imposes no strain on the system. And this is as true today as it was proved to be nearly forty years ago, when the first cell injection was performed. Indeed, these injections may be used where surgery is out of the question. On that first occasion they saved the patient's life.

Like many great scientific and medical discoveries the Niehans' method of cell therapy was the result of an accident.

The story goes back to a day in 1931. A young surgeon-pupil of Dr. de Quervain, then director of a well-known clinic in Lausanne, was operating on a woman patient for goiter when he accidentally cut her parathyroid glands.

Removal of the parathyroid glands produces tetany; a deep cut and removal, as was the case here, causes death within hours. The patient soon showed the characteristic muscular spasm of tetany and it was clear that if something drastic was not done quickly she would die.

Dr. de Quervain, called in by the young surgeon and his frightened theater staff, made the only life-saving decision possible: an immediate implant of animal parathyroids. But it had to be done very quickly; and even if it were possible to find and slaughter a suitable animal to provide the needed glands, there was the question of finding someone to perform the very delicate implant, which can often take an expert surgeon considerable time. This patient had perhaps two hours to live.

Suddenly de Quervain recalled the name of Paul Niehans, the author of a book on animal grafting which had recently been published, and was causing a stir in the medical world.

Niehans lived nearby in Montreux. The situation was desperate. De Quervain insisted that the brilliant but controversial doctor should be found at once and asked to do the grafting. . . .

Once located, Niehans lost no time in reaching the clinic. In readiness for the operation he had equipped himself with the parathyroid glands of a newly-born steer calf, but one glance at the patient convinced him that it was far too late to start operating. The case seemed hopeless.

Niehans, however, refused to be beaten. In his anxiety to save not only the patient's life but also the reputation of the young surgeon responsible for the initial mistake, he decided on a step he had never taken before.

Paul Niehans was, above all, an individualist. For some years he had been following his own line in research and building himself an impressive reputation for glandular grafting, that is to say, transplanting animal glands on to human beings.

[23]

In this he was following the work of Dr. Serge Voronoff of "monkey gland" fame; and he had already performed well over a thousand operations, including a delicate piece of brain surgery for the transfer of the anterior lobe of the pituitary gland of a calf to a human dwarf. This daring operation had yielded a spectacular result; the dwarf's height increased by one foot.

As if in a sudden flash of inspiration Niehans seized the gland that had been prepared for transplantation and, in his words, "cut it into very small pieces."

He said: "I put the pieces, together with a physiological serum, into a hypodermic syringe and injected the mixture into the patient's muscles connecting the arm and the chest."

The immediate results were striking and gratifying. Not only did the dreaded (and justifiably expected) anaphylactic shock, caused by the introduction of foreign protein, fail to set in, but within minutes the muscular cramps of tetany quietened down and then ceased.

Dr. Quervain, who had been expecting the patient's death at any moment, did not know what to think.

The patient was kept under close observation. Niehans stood by to give further injections in case of relapse. He said: "I thought at the time that the effects would be of short duration and that the injection would have to be repeated often to keep her alive." The theater staff stood by for what everyone believed would be the forthcoming big operation, the grafting of further parathyroid glands.

But the patient showed no signs of relapse; day by day her condition improved until, gradually, the truth began to dawn on the surgeons: they recognized with amazement that no glandular transplant operation would be necessary;

that the patient's constantly improving condition was not a temporary interlude but a permanent recovery; that in answer to a life-and-death challenge, Niehans had seemingly stumbled on a revolutionary new healing technique —the injection of animal cells into the human organism.

Although the revelation seemed to open up vast new horizons, it soon became clear that those horizons were in fact far distant, and the paths leading to them beset with every kind of difficulty.

In the first place, before attempting to go ahead with cell injections, there still remained a number of problems to be faced in connection with gland grafting; solutions to these were needed before a technique for cell therapy could be established.

One problem lay in the fact that few glandular grafts really "took"—that is to say, united with the tissue to which they were surgically joined. Also, it was noticed, in the few cases where the ingrafted tissue did take, the results were short-lived and that most were accompanied by violent allergic reactions.

It was not until the end of 1931 that Niehans discovered, by practical tests, that the answer to these problems lay in grafting from only newly-born or fetal animals. When this was done it was noticed that the ingrafted material was easily tolerated and that the patient's allergic reaction or anaphylactic shock was eliminated.

But for a long time after his discovery of cell therapy, Niehans cautiously concentrated on injecting tetany cases only, always with some degree of success and without allergic reaction, thanks to the uses of parathyroid cells from unborn or newly-born animals. It was only gradually that he extended the new technique to other cases, using other glands and non-glandular organs minced up, where formerly he would have performed transplant operations.

The results were highly gratifying even though, being extremely cautious, Niehans limited his treatments for the most part to patients who had been given up as hopelessly incurable and "not long for this world." But many of these patients, after their cell injections, found themselves with a good deal longer life span than had been expected and also were better able to enjoy the extra time.

Paul Niehans has been called many things in the course of his career, some of them flattering, some of them not, but no one can deny that this Swiss-born doctor has brought an unusual breadth of vision and depth of understanding to his new-found therapy and its implications.

Before turning to medicine he read both philosophy and theology, first at the University of Berne, which was his birthplace, then at Nuremberg, Oxford, Berlin and back again in Berne, gathering degrees effortlessly in one seat of learning after another.

The university stage of his career followed a brief spell of military service in deference to Hohenzollern family tradition: he is a stepnephew of Kaiser Wilhelm II through his mother, Anna Kauffmann, who was the illegitimate half-sister of the Kaiser.

Again, at one stage, Niehans had been on the point of taking up the ministry, in the Lutheran Church, as his life's work. But here again something made him stop: the decision perhaps that the cure of souls alone was not quite his line, and that he could do more satisfying work looking after body and soul together.

Even after qualifying as a doctor at Zurich he seemed to find narrow specialization for its own sake inconsistent with his particular brand of intellectual curiosity. He held various hospital appointments at this time, specializing in one field after another, all seemingly unrelated—opthalmology, gynecology, urology, endocrinology.

The First World War saw him as an International Red Cross medical inspector of the camps for Allied prisoners in Austria and Hungary. He worked on similar missions in the Second World War. All this experience tended to sharpen a growing desire to get to grips with some of the more depressing problems of existence like the remote causes of suffering and disease, degeneration, old age and decay.

A combination of his interests in endocrinology and surgery had early drawn Niehans' attention, as already mentioned, to the work of Serge Voronoff, the Russian-born naturalized Frenchman who was making his name through his efforts to revitalize the aged by grafting into them glands from young animals, especially monkeys.

The idea had not, of course, originated with Voronoff: it just happened to become surgically possible in his time. Medical history back through the ages to ancient Egypt and earlier is full of references to the use and efficiency of human and animal organs as healing or strengthening agents. To take a few of them: about 1400 B.C. Susruta, a famous Indian Guru and doctor, was prescribing tiger's blood and testes as a cure for debility and impotence; Achilles, the hero of Homer's Iliad, ate bone marrow from lions to gain their strength and prowess; a powder believed to be compounded of dried animal organs and spices has come down to us from Hippocrates, the fifth century B.C. "father" of modern medicine; human placenta, bull's blood, deer horn, fried spiders and tarantulas and similar organic

[27]

preparations were recommended as tonics and aphrodisiacs by Chinese doctors many centuries before the Christian era. Organic animal preparations figure prominently in the Materia Medica of Aristotle (384-322 B.C.) and of Pliny the Elder (A.D. 23-79).

The Swiss doctor-alchemist Paracelsus (Theophrastus Bombastus von Hohenheim, 1493-1541) coined the phrase *Similia similibus curentur,* meaning "treat like with like." A diseased organ, he explained, should be treated by administering the same organ from a healthy animal in dried or extracted form: heart for heart, kidney for kidney, and so on. An eighteenth-century list of medicines in use in Austria (compiled by Winkler in 1765) included 122 organic and glandular preparations, with contributions from the organs of executed criminals and burned witches.

It is one thing to drink the dried extract of human or animal organs as medicine; it is quite another thing, and a far better one, to have those organs, or their cells, young and vigorous, literally incorporated where they are needed, or so medical science has been thinking for the past two centuries at least. William Harvey, the English physician who discovered the circulation of the blood, seems to have been the first to put theory into practice, and with some degree of success. He transplanted the testes of a cock to a capon, and, for a short time, the capon became a cock again. (In parenthesis one can only marvel that the bird survived this piece of vivisection at all.)

With the introduction of anesthetics the number of similar attempts greatly increased. Operations were performed on both animals and human beings. They sought to implant animal tissue into animals and tissue from one human being to another. Some of the grafts were from adult to adult and were successful even in those days, though we do not know for how long. For example, in 1906 a surgeon named Morris transplanted human ovaries to a castrated woman who three years later gave birth to a child. Dartigues, in Paris, having removed an ovary from a patient, implanted it, for experimental purposes, into a previously castrated chimpanzee which then began to menstruate and later had young. The Italian Comoli in 1925 removed a parathyroid gland from a girl suffering from goiter and successfully implanted it to a woman suffering from tetany. In 1931 Dolby transferred the pancreas glands of newly stillborn infants to diabetics. The last operation, using cells instead of the whole gland, is normal treatment for diabetes mellitus at Dr. V. Schenks' clinic in Bremen, where stillborn pancreas glands are collected for the purpose from hospitals all over the Federal German Republic.

A similar scheme, but not yet socialized in application, is possible in Britain through the enterprise of a research group at the Royal Marsden Hospital in London, where a frozen embryonic tissue bank was established in 1959. Hospitals in any part of Britain may draw on this bank just as they do on frozen blood banks. Conservative and secretive though medical research workers notoriously are, especially in Britain, some early results of the work of this experimental tissue grafting and cell injecting did become known. The following extract is taken from a report which appeared in the *Daily Express* and other national newspapers on August 1, 1959:

A tiny thyroid gland taken from a small embryo will grow when transplanted to the adult human body. So will embryo liver, kidney and pieces of artery. The human body rapidly destroys such tissues when they are transplanted from another adult, or even from a child; but for some unknown reason embryo tissue is allowed to survive and grow.

Certain cells derived from premature stillborn babies can live and grow when injected into an adult human body. They are capable of replacing, and so to some extent revitalizing, tissues worn out through sickness or old age.

When simply injected into the blood stream of an adult,* embryo bone marrow cells will seek out the adult bone marrow, settle down there and multiply.

The year before these startling reports appeared, the general public were somewhat puzzled to read newspaper accounts of the emergency treatment that saved the lives of some Yugoslav atomic research workers who had been accidentally exposed to lethal doses of radiation. The injured were said to have been flown to Paris where they received *grafts* of bone marrow in operations at the Marie Curie Institute. No explanation of what was to be understood by the word "grafts" was given. And the ordinary layman could well have asked how a patient in an advanced state of leukemia could survive the surgeon's saw or gimlet hacking or boring through his bones. And which bones?

---

* All cell therapy injections are intramuscular, not intravenous.

[30]

Everyone knows that any surgical operation throws a great strain on the whole system, and that for this reason the patient needs considerable reserve vitality to draw on. Also, when the body's first line of defense—the blood—is broken down it is unreasonable to give it the additional task of repairing bone, tissue and skin, not to mention throwing off toxic effects of anesthesia.

But the fact was that the injured Yugoslav scientists recovered rapidly because they had received *injections* of bone-marrow cells: in other words, cell therapy. The use of the word "graft" to describe the measures taken in their case is simply an example of words in general circulation not having caught up with the facts of current practice. In the non-scientific vocabulary of everyday life, the older word often sticks illogically despite its obvious misuse. And this was indeed the explanation here. In other words, cell injections had been given where surgical operation was out of the question, and successfully.

However, the big problem for many years to come was how to make the cells readily available everywhere, and as easily prepared for injection and administration as vaccines and serums. Cells separated from the connective tissue of their parent organism—for example, pancreas cells isolated from the pancreas, liver cells isolated from the liver—do not live for more than two or three hours at the most. Niehans abandoned the search for a formula for a preparation of isolated cells only when he had nearly killed himself in an experiment in 1949. As always his own chief guinea pig, he gave himself a shot of several days' old frozen cell solution warmed to body temperature. In one of his books he has described how he quickly be-

[31]

came dizzy, nauseated, and lapsed into unconsciousness before he was able to get out of his laboratory.

This near-fatal experiment proved that freezing cannot prevent cells in solution from becoming toxic after a time. Some other means of cell viability had to be found if the treatment was not to be restricted to those who could afford to have it in nursing homes or clinics with specially supervised animal farms and slaughtering establishments attached; exactly, in fact, what Niehans has at his clinic near Vevey on Lake Geneva.

The next trial method of cell preparation was rapid deep freezing after extraction of moisture. This proved satisfactory in some 6,000 experimental injections, first into animals and then into human beings. Still there was room for improvement. To get the deep-frozen cells to all parts of the world would be costly and not always practicable, since their transport would require specially insulated containers. So the search went on for the ideal cell preparation, one in which the cells would retain their potency independent of time and place.

There is a difference between moisture extraction and dehydration; that difference held the elusive possibilities sought in vain by other means. Complete dehydration so that the live cells became a dry powder has been found to be the answer to the problem of safe cell viability dissociated from connective tissue. The cells are reconstituted for liquid injection and may be stored like any other pharmaceutical product. After thorough investigation of the whole matter and of Niehans' private experiments, a leading pharmaceutical firm in Germany has for some years been producing a dry cell powder in sealed ampules, and another independent firm is now taking over the production of cell matter. When reconstituted in a special saline solution the dried cells are said to be exactly the same as fresh ones, and, in fact, may be observed under the microscope quivering, splitting and multiplying. Further more, their use eliminates the element of danger through negligence attendant, however remotely, upon the introduction of fresh cells into the human body. Dried cells are always preferred by Niehans in cases of old age and debility where the fresh cells, in his opinion, could be too stimulating. And they are always used for cell therapy injections in Britain and in other clinics throughout the world.

3

The Cell

To understand the potential value of cell therapy it is necessary, first of all, to know something about the cell itself, and a little, too, of its relationship to the human system.

Put simply, the cell is the source of the body's life and energy in the same way that a spring or a well is a source of water.

Healthy cells, especially those of the unborn or the newly-born, and whether of human or animal origin, are endowed with a super-abundance of energy or life force. Each cell, as it divides and multiplies, passes on this energy to every pair of new cells, so that each new pair, possesses, or should possess, the same amount of vital energy as the parent cell.

When we are in good health all our cells are in a constant state of replacement and renewal. This process is essential to sustain life; in fact, it *is* life.

[34]

But with the cell it is quality that counts. Everything depends on the quality of the renewed cells because in the long run quality will affect the quantity, too.

In a young growing organism the cells multiply far in excess of replacement needs. The excess constitutes the process of growth.

In a healthy adult the excess, though slight, is still sufficient to ensure a supply of newly-born cells to meet emergency repair needs in cases of illness or accident.

A disease of the body, then, must stem from a disease of its cells. Long before we realize that we are ill, our cells have been in a bad state. And by the time the symptoms are bad enough to call for treatment, weak, diseased cells have been dying off far in excess of replacement. Somewhere along the line, in the chain reaction of cell replacement the weak links have crept in; and often much too early in life we begin to feel perpetually tired, never really well enough to enjoy life as we used to enjoy it and we feel, while we struggle to keep up appearances, that we have the right to enjoy it.

It is a fact that the stress and strain of modern life contribute substantially to this loss of vital energy at its source. Nevertheless it is important, in assessing the value of cell therapy, to remember the chain reaction of cell renewal, precisely because, as we have already said, each new pair of cells possesses the same amount of vital energy as the parent cell.

Some biologists consider that as the strong, healthy cell approaches the end of its life's cycle—which can vary from a few hours to the body's lifetime—it secretes a hormone that stimulates the birth of its successor.

[35]

This is a reasonable theory. The cause of the death of the whole organism is due to the fact that as the organism ages there is an increase in the production of mutated cells which are not destroyed by the body's defense mechanism. Weak, unhealthy cells cannot give birth to strong healthy ones, and when these weak sickly cells die by the million and are replaced by similar sickly cells, then comes the time when the whole organism—the human body—can no longer be maintained in life.

But the will to live, plus—as we shall show in the following pages—*the excess vitality in the cells of the unborn or newly born of other species,* can save the degenerate human system before this stage is reached.

This, in a nutshell, is what cell therapy is about.

To deal with human diseases, failing health or loss of vitality on the level of the cell is to get right down to fundamentals: it is to harness the "nuclear energy" of the cell in the interest of individual repair and recovery. (The expression "nuclear energy," applied to the cell, is no metaphor but sober fact.)

Cytology, the study of the cell, is one of the youngest of the biological sciences. It has been able to profit from the use of the electron microscope, radioactive tracer elements and other contemporary technical devices. Recent research on the subject shows that the inexplicable phenomenon of life force, or the will to live, comes from the nucleus of the cell and works with a blind tenacious energy to surmount all obstacles in fulfilling its purpose, the particular purpose laid down for the cell by Nature in her master plan. But what exactly is a cell? The textbook definition is that it is a unit of physiological activity, a working area for the microscopic bodies within. Bodies, microscopic or otherwise, working purposefully together as a unit, constitute a highly organized society, and the cell has been rightly compared to a state within a state—the organism it serves.

Leading cytologists tend to the view that the energy or life force in each cell and the way it is used are the results of chemical reaction.

Severo Ochoa, an American medical biologist who won the 1959 Nobel Prize jointly with his fellow countryman, Arthur Kornberg, for their work on cell nuclei, has written: "All life is chemistry, the more we get to know and are able to prove about the chemical reactions of the cells the closer we shall approach the phenomenon of life itself."

In the nuclei of living cells biologists have isolated two substances which they believe to be responsible for chemical reactions of life processes. These substances are: deoxyribonucleic acid and ribonucleic acid. The first, DNA, is the nearest we can get, materially, to the life force that carries on the species; the second, RNA, is the nearest we can get to a material explanation of the differences between individuals.

In man and the higher animals, life begins with a single fertilized cell, the ovum. In the human embryo it grows into a being composed eventually of some forty trillion cells, the brain alone having nine billion nerve cells, or neurons. The growth process is by division into identical units, the first cell becoming two, the two becoming four, and so on; followed by a highly complex system of differentiation for specialization. The nucleus of the fertilized cell contains the genetic pattern of the unborn creature according to his species, the detailed plan of the individual characteristics that will distinguish him from his fellows, and a directional center (the "primary organizer") to control the working out of the pattern in the orderly system of growth that we take for granted. The two nucleic acids, DNA and RNA, are the key chemical executives in charge of the whole process.

Every cell in the human body has its preordained purposes to fulfill. This is the reason for the change-over in the developing embryo from a system of duplication of identical cells to one of differentiation, in which each new pair of cells has a specific building function and location. The cells of every organ and tissue have their distinctive chemical composition and type of protein. How this process of differentiation happens is something that science has yet to discover. The French biologist, Minot, has suggested that if we understood the process of cell differentiation we should have solved the mystery of life itself.

Ribonucleic acids control the synthesis of proteins specific to each organ in primary growth and, afterwards, in maintenance by cell renewal throughout life. They are thus in charge of the development of all those small differences that distinguish one individual from another—the inherited genetic characteristics of physical make-up and otherwise, including all kinds of irregularities and susceptibilities to various disorders. RNA is not self-sufficient however, but derives its powers, so to speak, from DNA, for the two chief nucleic acids are complementary and interdependent. DNA is known to be the basis of all life. Even the most elementary of self-reproducing parasitic organisms like the virus have DNA in their chemical composition. It is present in the human genes which pass on the architectural plan of characteristics inherited from the parents, and some of those that the parents in their turn have themselves inherited. Some scientists maintain that the genes, of which the human organism has about 40,000, consist entirely of DNA.

In DNA there are four elementary substances: Cytosin, Adenin, Guanin and Thymin, which must be present in the appropriate order. So long as that natural chemical construction remains unchanged, individuals and species remain the same. If, however, nature errs, or human interference upsets the strict order of these basic elements, a mutation occurs, causing not only inheritable individual peculiarities, but intrinsic changes in the species.

The other leading nucleic acid, RNA, also contains four basic elements. They are Cytosin, Guanin, Adenin and Uracil. They, too, must occur strictly in the appropriate order to form specific proteins for organ building, since RNA is "organotrope," that is to say, concerned with specific organs, RNA for kidneys builds only kidney protein; RNA for liver forms liver protein only, and so on. Like DNA, RNA multiplies by an automatic process, the secret of which may be explained by what is known as the template theory. Thus the cell obeys a life force which human science fails to understand, is unable to imitate or synthetize; it is ruled by laws of nature which we have only just begun to grasp.

Experiments without number, for instance, have proved the all but indestructible quality of the life force of cells in groups outside the body. One of the most remarkable biological experiments of the twentieth century was that of the French scientist, Alexis Carrel, who wanted to find out how long a group of cells would remain alive outside the body to which they had belonged. He put fragments from the heart of a chicken embryo into nourishing plasma

[39]

in an incubator. For the first sixty-five days nothing appeared to be happening, but on the sixty-sixth day the heart fragments began to show a rhythmic pulsating movement. When placed together the fragments at once began to unite and to grow together. The whole then moved in one rhythmic heart beat. Carrel kept his piece of chicken heart alive for thirty-four years, that is, for more than eighty chicken generations, and for years after the death of the embryo which had been the owner of the heart. There were no signs of aging or degeneration in the group of cells which, to all appearances, could have gone on living for ever.

Carrel also observed, experimentally, the healing effect of healthy cells on the unhealthy. A group of cells taken from a diseased animal and kept in nourishing plasma in an incubator showed litle sign of life until a quantity of healthy young animal cells were added. Some time after this addition the entire group of cells was seen to be in good condition and reproducing normally.

It has often been demonstrated that the destruction of an embryo does not destroy the life of its component cells. Animal embryos have been cut up, minced and passed through fine sieves, and their cell groups have remained unharmed. With the encouragement of warmth and nourishment (incubator and suitable plasma) they grew healthily and remained young. The most drastic experiments of this kind have been carried out on cells both before and after they had reached the phase of differentiation.

Hans Spemann, a 1935 Nobel Prize winner for Physiology and Medicine, made some amazing discoveries about severed cell groups before differentiation, that is, when all the cells in an embryo are exactly the same. He found that when a scrap of embryo skin is implanted into a nerve of the same embryo it grows and behaves like a nerve; similarly, when nerve cells are grafted into the epidermic regions they grow like and become skin. This demonstrates that at the pre-differential stage cells are identical and interchangeable. They can serve all purposes in the developing organism to which they belong and, as we shall presently see, all purposes in any other organism of the same molecular structure as themselves. In other words, the life force in the cell is so strong it cannot easily be thwarted; it will combine with any suitable material in order to live and grow.

The opposite phenomenon—the determination of specialized, differentiated cells to carry out their genetic instructions despite all obstacles—has been demonstrated by Doctor Paul Weiss and A. Cecil Taylor of the Rockefeller Institute, who described striking experiments of this nature in the 1959 proceedings of the United States Academy of Natural Sciences. They took various small parts of several chicken embryos between one and two weeks old, that is, when the stage of differentiation in a chicken embryo is past. They minced up the fragments as finely as possible, separating the cells with enzymes containing DNA and RNA. From this mash containing millions of cells destined to form various organs they implanted minute traces of the membrane, or sack, enclosing the eight to fourteen-day-old chicken embryos. After some incubation time, during which they were nourished by the membrane's own blood supply, the implanted cells organized themselves again and began to grow.

Liver cells developed into a minute liver, one-sixth of an inch long and capable of purifying the blood of a nonexistent chicken on the same scale. Kidney cells formed

[41]

an infinitely tiny kidney. Skin cells became a tiny section of skin which sprouted feathers one-tenth of an inch long. All the cells in fact tried to complete their original tasks according to the master plan of the vanished embryo to which they had belonged.

Superficially, ducks and mice appear to have nothing in common. Etienne Wolff proved the contrary when he succeeded in uniting pieces of liver taken from newly born specimens of the two species. Because they had the same molecular structure, the pieces tolerated each other and grew together as a unit. This is a basic law of nature. The urge to live and grow is so strong that, removed from their parent organism, cells will integrate with an organism outside their own species, provided the molecular structure of the alien organism is the same as their own.

But this tolerance only occurs if the ingrafted cells or tissue are very young, preferably fetal or newly born.

Genetic differentiation makes every adult different in structural and chemical detail. For this reason the cells and tissues of adults do not tolerate one another; and for the same reason we hear of the failure of efforts to transplant a kidney, a liver or a heart from one adult to another, while, in the case of a successful skin graft, the grafted skin is always taken from another part of the patient's own body. The exceptions are identical twins, (triplets, quadruplets, etc.) who, genetically, are one person. Their RNA is identical.

This, then, is the essence of cell therapy, or biological repair to the human organism: a therapy which consists in taking advantage in the first place of the mutual tolerance of cells and tissues with the same molecular structure, though belonging to a totally different species, and, in the

[42]

second place, of the tremendous hardihood of healthy cells which gives them an indomitable energy (that mysterious life force which is the "will to live") in overcoming all obstacles to growth within their own molecular structure.

Surprising though it may seem to many people, it is a fact that domestic animals such as pigs, sheep and calves are of the same molecular structure as human beings; consequently there is a natural affinity between their cells and those of the human organism.

The superabundant vitality of the young animal, preferably the fetus, specially bred and selected, can restore and rebuild the flagging life force in human beings. Cellular therapy uses this discovery therapeutically for human regeneration.

4

How Cell Therapy Works

MANY theories have been advanced to explain what happens to cells injected into the human body and how their therapeutical effects are produced. Taken together the known facts lead to one conclusion: cells by their nature are forever trying to carry on the impulse and pattern of embryonic development, that is to say, to unite with others of their kind, multiply and build up into their predetermined whole. To do this they have to move: indeed movement is one of the chief characteristics of cell behavior: under a microscope embryo cells can be seen moving at the rate of half an inch an hour.

It is not definitely known whether the whole cells, as injected, travel inside the body, or only some of their components. But it is possible to trace the progress of groups of cells which have been dyed before injection. Experiments have shown that the routes taken by the injected cells—seen by means of the dye as fine lines radiating in various directions from the site of injection—are clearly discernible for four days only. After that it is believed that the cells disintegrate, releasing their components—the vital nucleic acids and proteins—to find their way by chemical attraction to the sites where they are needed. This is one theory.

Another has it that the injected cells continue to live in the muscle at the injection site. There the capillaries nourish them and provide them with oxygen, transporting only their secretions through the blood stream.

Chemotherapy is based on precisely this principle of teleaction. For example, medicines taken into the stomach are expected to benefit, and do benefit, other parts of the body which have no direct connection with the process of elimination. The principle is taken for granted in all routine medical injections and inoculations: whether it is the whole body or just part of it that is to be benefited, the injected material enters by an arm, a leg or a buttock.

A variant, then, of this same idea is that the injected cells disintegrate at or around the injection site, and that their components travel to the appropriate organ, or area, to be used as repair material. Radiation has shown this to be true of injections into animals. Lettre, of Heidelberg, radioactivated the components of a group of animal cells, injected them into a test animal and traced the injected material to a distant group of cells that had become radioactive. His theory is that it is the infinitely small and complicated parts of a cell known as mitochondria which are the chief active agents in cell injection.

But whether the cells reach their target area whole or broken down, their specific action on that area is a proven fact. Two German medical biologists, Dr. Dittman, of

Hoxter, and Dr. Neumann, of Cologne, injected very small, young animals with specific cells and found that the organs and glands at which the therapy was aimed developed more quickly and showed a greater increase in size than untreated organs and glands.

Given, then, the natural urge of cells to move, and the fact that the human body consists of about 90 percent fluid, including the ever-moving blood cells, it would be surprising if injected cells and their chemical components remained static. To carry out their functions, the body's own cells are in a state of near perpetual motion, and in cases of emergency, such as accident or illness, they may be sent anywhere required. This is so because throughout life the cell growth pattern laid down in the embryo continues, or perhaps it would be safer to say, *tries* to continue. The pattern, as mentioned earlier, is one of multiplication by division into, first, undifferentiated cells capable of taking on any building-repair job anywhere and the differentiated cells for the maintenance and repair of specific organs and glands.

In ideal conditions, whole armies of undifferentiated cells would be available for the rebuilding of tissue damaged in an accident; also for emergency replacements for differentiated cells in an organ undermined by infection or disease, when the organ's own rate of cell replacement becomes grossly inadequate and needs help from somewhere, within or without. In the conditions in which most people live today, little emergency help is available from within; there are hardly any reserves of vitality to draw on. (Vitality, or life force, as explained in the last chapter, is healthy cell production somewhat in excess of day-to-day needs. That other vitality, by which we vaguely mean plenty of energy and high spirits, is also directly due to having healthy cells and a few to spare.)

In chronic illness and degenerative processes the body's power of cell reproduction is the first thing to suffer. Quality goes first: the cell's precious neucleic components, including DNA and RNA without which no living thing as we know it would exist, are greatly weakened. It is not surprising that in this state the human body rapidly accepts help from outside in the form of vital young cells from other species, provided these are embryonic or newly-born and therefore will not provoke any allergic antagonisms or anaphylactic shock. These new cells revive and reinforce the body's own powers of cell renewal, starting off a chain reaction of strong, healthy cell production.

And this boost can be passed on. In matters of personal health people are often too shortsighted and self-centered to give a thought to posterity, although they are always affronted if they find that their children or grandchildren are physically or mentally below their expectations—sometimes even deficient. But by means of cell therapy, when large amounts of new and vigorous DNA and RNA stimulate old, tired or diseased tissues so that they begin to reproduce with renewed vitality, the newly acquired additional life force manifested in the improved quality of each renewed cell is then passed on to the new generations of healthier individuals. Thus not only the individual receiving the cell injections but the family, indeed the species, can all benefit.

It may be as well at this point to refute some of the popular fallacies existing in relation to cell therapy. First, the cells of another species—lamb, calf, pig—used therapeutically do NOT transmit their individual characteristics, or those of their species, to human beings. Persons injected do NOT become bovine, sheeplike or piggish.

In 1889 a scientist named Brown-Sequard made a sterilized aqueous extract of dog's testes and injected himself with it subcutaneously. He declared the result to be stimulating and rejuvenating, but he did NOT begin to bark and bite, and he did not beget pups.

Voronoff's famous monkey gland operations inspired many a music hall skit and private joke, but the assumption, however facetious, that a patient grafted with tissue from a monkey thereafter acted like one simply had no foundation in fact. The laws of genetics are against such a possibility. The rare patient who was *successfully* grafted with an animal gland experienced a pleasant sense of enhanced vitality and well-being which, alas, was short-lived. . . . But grafting by cell injection is an advance on this older method of tissue grafting by surgery. Apart from the obvious advantages in avoiding surgery, it is biologically sounder, more sensitive, gentler, subtler and more pervasive in its action.

Another mistaken assumption about cell therapy—due to sensational misrepresentation in the popular press—is that it produces a miraculous rejuvenation. In fact it does not. In any case the word is wrongly used: there is no such thing as rejuvenation, since *true physiological rejuvenation* would involve a reversal of the laws of Nature—a growing younger every day instead of older until we were finally back in the cradle and the womb.

The word "revitalization" is a truer description of what takes place following cell therapy: and this process of revitalization can and does achieve *functional rejuvenation,* which is what the sensation-mongers really mean.

[48]

Aging is a fact, a natural process, a cosmic law. There are some fortunate people who age very, very slowly, so that to their friends they never seem to grow any older. But there are also others—the vast majority—who age rapidly and prematurely. And these are the people cell therapy can help. In such people the physiological and mental processes of aging can be reversed to a point *natural and normal to that individual were he living in more ideal conditions.*

So the tired middle-aged man or woman, suffering from physical and mental decline, disease and degeneration, does not look 25 again after treatment, but is made to feel different, healthier and happier. In these circumstances he and she forget their age, and because they no longer worry about it, actually do look younger. The injection of new life contained in the young cells not only triumphs over their ill-health but infuses the whole flagging system with the vitality it lacked before.

Indispensable in successful treatment by cell therapy is expert diagnosis of the patient's condition. And here routine medical examination with the usual clinic tests is often not enough. A searching system of scientifically accurate diagnosis has been worked out by the German biochemist Professor Emile Abderhalden.

The Abderhalden resistance-ferment reaction tests are so called because they record and measure a certain type of ferment which is formed in the organs and glands and excreted in the urine whenever the normal function of any gland or organ is disturbed. Each gland and organ has its own distinctive ferment. Test results not only reveal incipient dysfunction of glands and organs not detectable by ordinary diagnostic methods but also to what degree they may be dysfunctioning, diseased or decaying. If no specific ferment can be found in the urine this means the organ being investigated is either healthy or nonexistent because it has been removed by operation. Such a system of diagnosis is naturally laborious and complicated, and requires extremely elaborate equipment. So far there are only three laboratories in the world where the Abderhalden diagnostic tests can be made. They are in Basle, Cologne and Barcelona.

There are not many single, straightforward diseases or causes of ill-health, since one deficiency sooner or later leads to others, and treatment often has to be given for a whole series of dysfunctions. No good practitioner treats a single defective organ but the entire human being.

Generally speaking, in all cases of organic underfunction or age-conditioned organic degeneration, the corresponding animal cells (always fetal or newly born) are administered. The same treatment applies in cases of glandular underfunction or degeneration, with the administration of the corresponding animal gland cells. If a gland is overfunctioning, however, its antagonist must be activated. The antagonist, or inhibitor, of a gland is another gland which has partly or completely the opposite action. If, for example, the pituitary gland in an older patient is overactive (as often happens), cells of its antagonist, the pineal gland, or gonads, or other target glands are injected. (The pineal gland is used after experiments in cell therapy rather than in general physiology.) Increased activity of the pineal curtails the activity of the pituitary. Some glands are sex-conditioned and are thus administered according to the sex of the patient.

In cases of excessive degeneration through old age, or

where long illness has undermined the whole organism, it is often necessary to administer a large variety of cell preparations in substantial quantities. Such treatments have to be spread over several sessions to avoid excessive stress for the patient, especially if it is a case of marked general debility. When, however, the general condition of the patient is fairly satisfactory, and not too many injections are required, all the injections may be given in a single session. Cells of separate organs have to be injected separately. When large amounts of cells of one kind have to be injected, possibly in an attempt to achieve a quick result, the total quantity may be administered at two sites. The site of the injection is always the seat or buttocks —except in the cases of bone fracture, when bone cells are injected locally.

To obtain the full benefit from treatment it is important that the patient, even a fairly healthy one, should stay in bed for at least three days following injection. If treatment is given in two or more sessions the patient stays in bed for three days after each. During the two weeks following treatment no drugs, laxatives, sleeping tablets or any other medicine may be taken unless prescribed by the practitioner. Any drug may counteract or delay the effects of the injected cells; large doses of drugs, especially the sulfa group, may render a cell treatment totally ineffective. For some time after injection the patient must abstain from nicotine, alcohol, undue physical exertion, X rays, sources of radiation, diathermy, shortwave treatment, excessive hot or cold baths, Turkish baths and sunbathing. The one indulgence permitted is the consumption of vitamins; sufficient of these, especially vitamin C, may be taken.

Only in cases of infectious diseases such as pneumonia, meningitis, tuberculosis, venereal diseases and all other conditions caused by bacteria and viruses is cell therapy not indicated. The reason is that in such cases the infection would destroy the new cells. When the infection has been eliminated, cell therapy can be very beneficial in restoring lost vitality and repairing the damage done by the infection.

5

The Glands

In sketching this overall picture of cell therapy, reference has frequently been made to glands. These are mainly the endocrine glands, organs of internal secretion which pour their particular product directly into the blood stream, and whose balanced activity is essential to the maintenance of physical and mental health.

This chapter will discuss some of the more important glands, explain their functions briefly and show how cell therapy can correct glandular imbalance, the source of many, often seemingly inexplicable, organic disorders.

Hidden away in various parts of the body, the endocrine glands all have partners, each complementary to the other and all interdependent, which means that if one is out of order then, sooner or later, the rest are affected.

Imagine a magnificient orchestra with the bass-cello coming in on the wrong note and the clarinets constantly playing out of tune. The other performers do what they can to cover up, but this means that they also are playing slightly off-beat, with too great a volume of sound in the wrong places, increased tempo and so on. If the process is allowed to continue unchecked, the music becomes chaos, and, of course, it is agony for the conductor. Substitute "endocrine glands" for "the orchestra" and "owner of the glands" for "the conductor" and you have a pretty clear picture of quite a common state of affairs.

In the case of the orchestra the conductor can in the last resort change his musicians. In the case of the endocrine glands, however, substitution is not so easy. It is true that replacement surgery may be resorted to in an emergency, and, provided the implanted glands have come from a human or animal embryo, with some hope of success for the patient, after a long and difficult period of adjustment. But the proceduce necessarily throws a considerable strain on the whole system and, in the case of some deep-seated glands in the body, can constitute a very grave risk. In other words, the finest surgery in the world is still a crude and drastic way of dealing with glandular disorder.

Hormone treatment—the internal secretions of the ductless glands are called hormones—superseded the risky glandular grafting but even hormone therapy has turned out to be nothing more than a rather clumsy effort at doing for a gland what it apparently cannot do for itself.

The classic example is the treatment of diabetes mellitus with injections of insulin, the hormone which the pancreas gland should supply in sufficient quantities for itself. As is usual in hormone treatment, the insulin injections have often to continue for life. They do nothing to stimulate the defective gland into activity; on the contrary they encourage it to atrophy; and in the case of the diabetic patient, for instance, the endocrinologist must, in some cases, as time goes on, administer more and more of the synthetic hormone.

Most glands, however, do not secrete one straightforward hormone but a variety; also they stimulate their antagonists to produce each its own totally different set of hormones, and it is the combined effects of these that strike the happy glandular balance which adds up to good health.

The prolonged substitution of one synthetic hormone for a series of natural products has a thoroughly unbalancing effect, not only because each gland by its hormone production activates its antagonist; but also because when a gland is particularly inactive, its antagonist grows sluggish as well, and to counterbalance their combined shortcomings other glands must automatically work overtime.

It is not surprising, therefore, that endocrine disturbances are seldom simple but nearly always pluri- or multi-glandular.

Many organic disorders are merely the result of glandular dysfunction. But is is extremely difficult, even for an experienced endocrinologist, to decide which gland is over-functioning and which is underfunctioning the most, which one caused the primary disturbance and how many other glands have been affected in consequence. Diagnosis by the Abderhalden test method greatly reduces the possibility or error and uncertainty: because, by this method, whatever the condition of the glands, it shows up by the deposits of glandular ferments in the urine.

To take a hypothetical case: a patient suffering from obesity can be prescribed (by orthodox medicine) countless pills, slimming diets and thyroid tablets, and yet show no result or reaction other than palpitations and nervous irritability cause by the thyroid tablets. A standard medical prescription of thyroid for obesity simply does not work in this case.

But the Abderhalden tests may reveal quite a different seat of glandular disturbance—the pituitary. And this is where cell therapy can be very effective; for when the patient is treated with injections of pituitary cells he begins steadily to lose weight and eventually he will look normal again.

This hypothetical case is, of course, oversimplified: pituitary dysfunctions rarely occur alone. As already pointed out, endocrine disturbances are almost invariably pluri- or multi-glandular. Treatment by cell therapy will call for substantial quantities of cell injections for the most disturbed gland (or, if that gland is overfunctioning, for its antagonist); and small quantities of appropriate cells will be given for the other affected glands. For example, cells of the hypothalamus are likely to be included, for in nearly all glandular dysfunctions the hypothalamus is found to be debilitated to some degree.

Certain glands have key roles in the human chemical works. *The pituitary* is one of these. It is undoubtedly the most important central station for the body's entire hormone production, exercising as it does a harmonizing influence on all other ductless glands. The list of its 24 known hormones is not necessarily complete; and although much has recently been learned about this gland and its influence, there still remains a good deal to be explained.

The pituitary produces ACTH, a substance widely used in modern medicine, which has an anti-inflammatory, reaction-resisting influence. Pituitary cells are therefore included in cell treatments where the diagnosis indicates proneness to inflammation, all arthritic conditions, little resistance to extraneous infections, chronic catarrhs and various kinds of skin complaints.

When the separate parts of the pituitary either over- or under-function together with the target glands, results then show in abnormal increases in growth and weight, or in no increase at all; youngsters either grow to be giants or remain physically children greatly retarded mentally and retarded in sexual maturity. Adults with this type of glandular imbalance either become abnormally fat, or fail to put on any weight at all.

Underdevelopment of the pituitary may also inhibit the development of the thyroid, parathyroid, suprarenal glands or gonads.

Insufficient development of the latter causes impotence in the male, and amenorrhoea or menstruation difficulties in the female. In such cases, too—except where tumor or cancer is suspected—cells of one or more parts of the pituitary are injected.

Disturbances of the pituitary are frequent. During the male and female climacteric the pituitary gland is often found to be overactive. In that case the cells of its antagonist, the pineal gland, are among those injected.

When the target glands fail to exercise their braking influence, abnormal mental developments or sexual precociousness may occur at an early age. The results of this may be child prodigies, geniuses at school, but used up mentally and physically to the point of senility at the normal age of maturity. Underfunction of the target glands may produce tumors of various kinds. In all such cases cell injection of these glands are given.

The thyroid is another important gland: if it does not function sufficiently the production of thyroxin ceases or is reduced and brain activity slows down.

Signs of thyroid deficiency include general sluggishness, feeling cold without reason, decline in pulse rate, oedema (swelling) in the face and elsewhere, skin and hair in bad condition. Injections of thyroid cells will, in such cases, be included in the treatment.

Thyroid cells, with brain and other cells, are included in the treatment for mongolism, where brain activity must be stimulated. They are also given to reduce weight (when overweight is caused by thyroidal dysfunction), and with other cells, in cases of osteoarthritis, gout, impotence or sterility. When, together with thyroidal dysfunction, the parathyroids are overactive, calcium accumulates in the joints, arteries and brain. This is typical of the very prevalent condition known as arteriosclerosis, or hardening of the arteries. Thyroid and parathyroid cells are always included in the cell therapy for this condition.

Disturbance of the thyroid can occur at any age, quite suddenly, as the result of undue stress for any length of time, or of a mental nervous shock. And when this gland gets out of step it seldom puts itself right if left untreated.

Common signs of parathyroid underfunction are muscular cramps, aches and pains in the muscles, or headaches that feel like a ring round the head.

The thymus gland controls physical growth in childhood. Later, when no longer required as a store of building material for the growing body, it atrophies.

Thymus cells are included in the treatment of physically underdeveloped and mongoloid children. Thymus cells also prove beneficial in cases of premature aging, in states of exhaustion, after long illness, habitual abortion, and in some cases of cataract and arthritis.

When the pancreas gland goes on strike, glucose is no longer available for cellular activity but eliminated instead in the urine, and diabetes develops.

Since there can be about eight different causes of this complaint, it would not be correct to treat diabetes automatically with pancreas cells alone. When the diabetes is caused by damage to hypothalamus, gonads, kidney or liver, for instance, cells of these glands and organs usually contribute to a cure. And gonad cells are used when the diabetes is caused by overfunctioning of the pituitary and suprarenal glands, or by the underfunctioning of the gonads. In straightforward diabetes mellitus, however, the so-called Langerhans islets of the pancreas are disturbed and cell therapy consists largely of pancreas cells.

Human pancreas cells are most effective for the treatment of this condition. A German physician in Bremen, for instance, treats his diabetes mellitus with such cells derived from stillborn infants.

Although suprarenal glands have two parts with distinct characteristics and influence—the cortex, or upper layer, and the medulla, or inner body—their functions sometimes overlap.

Overfunction of the cortex causes oedema, abnormal hair growth on the face or body, and makes the sufferer feel constantly hot.

Underfunction of the cortex produces a sensation of coldness, unhealthy hair and nails, a feeling of tiredness and lack of energy. (This condition is often the result of alcohol, nicotine or drug addiction, and unless the patient stops his excesses, cell therapy will not have much effect.)

In treatment, cortex cells are indicated in cases of abnormal thinness, weakness, exhaustion, lack of energy, low resistance, unduly low blood pressure, bad circulation causing a permanent sensation of cold, arthritis, arthrosis, gout, baldness and poor hair. They are also indicated to improve the function of lungs, heart, liver and stomach.

The medulla of the suprarenal gland regulates the amount of adrenaline in the blood—adrenaline gives energy, increases blood pressure and improves breathing difficulties.

In treatment, these medulla cells are helpful in cases of low blood pressure and asthma. But they should not be given to persons suffering from certain heart complaints, high blood pressure or arteriosclerosis, with the danger of a stroke.

The cells of the gonads and the placenta are so important for health that they are always included in every cell treatment for their general tonic properties. Their influence on the human organism is so great, in fact, that any description of their effects soon shows where the "popular miracle cure" and "rejuvenation" stories surrounding cell therapy originated. . . .

The gonads—testes in the male and the ovaries in the female—are not only connected with sex and reproduction but produce numerous hormones which bring physical strength and energy, mental alertness and vitality. These glands are indeed a font of health and vigor and youth to the entire cell state and the whole human system. They also have a rejuvenating effect on the entire aging male system, bringing an improvement in circulation which has its effect on heart, tissues and all organs, normalizing blood pressure and imparting a better texture to skin and hair.

In treatment, testes cells are indicated for boys in cases of slow development and immaturity, bedwetting and effeminate development. For adults they are helpful in cases of impotence, various sexual neuroses, inferiority complexes and shyness, lack of circulation, arteriosclerosis, heart trouble, angina pectoris, chronic pulsating head-aches, dizziness, congestion, insomnia, several skin diseases and, last but not least, the male climacteric with its usual symptoms: decline in libido and potency, prostate disorders, decline in physical strength and resistance, depression and loss of self-confidence. In general, testes cells are given to aid all healing processes; and, according to Niehans, they have been proved to be a prophylaxis for cancer-endangered patients and to retard its development.

Ovary cells for women have effects similar to those of the testes for males. They are divided into two kinds: follicular cells and corpus luteum cells, and secrete two hormones; the follicular hormone (oestrone), and the hormone of the corpus luteum.

The secretions of the follicle cells give the essential feminine appearance and develop the breasts. They are given to girls who have not yet reached puberty and women after the climacteric; to the type of girl whose physical womanly development is retarded; as a cure for most menstruation troubles, such as amenorrhoea and dysmenorrhoea, sterility caused by menstruation disturbance and difficulty in lactation. They are also helpful in cases of anemia, overfunction of the thyroid, all troubles connected with the change of life, growth of bodily hair, rheumatism after the climacteric, arteriosclerosis, angina pectoris, high blood pressure, various skin diseases, premature aging, and, again according to Niehans, as a prophylaxis against cancer.

The placenta is the medium of nutrition for the developing embryo up to the time of birth, when it is discharged. It has everything required for growth. And its usefulness cannot be better confirmed than by recalling the well-known fact that mother animals, after giving birth to their young, eat their own placenta in an instinctive urge to benefit from the multitude of hormones, vitamins and other substances it contains.

The healing, reintegrating, rejuvenating and generally stimulating qualities of the placenta have been known since time immemorial and have always had a prominent place in folklore and folk medicine. Indeed, primitive peoples still use the placenta for various remedial purposes. And it is a fact that the truth and wisdom about the therapeutic value of natural substances handed down through the centuries in myths, legends, superstitions and old wives' tales are sometimes confirmed by scientific research and orthodox medical views. Never was this more clearly illustrated than by the return of scientific medicine to the use of the active healing properties and principles of the placenta.

The biological activity of the placenta is multiple and far-reaching. It is a factory and storage depot for a quantity of substances which have an extensive influence on the entire endocrine system and on all organs; hence placenta cells occupy a prominent place in cell therapy. The following is by no means an exhaustive list of substances found in the placenta, all vital for the formation, maintenance and functional rejuvenation of the human system.

Hormones: ACTH, Prolan, Oestron, Progesteron.
Vitamins: A, B, C, D, E.

Ferments: Diastases, Histaminases, Hyaluronidases, Lipases, Lactases, Saccharases, Phosphatases, Arginases, Peroxydases, Adenyl-pyrophosphatases, Amino-oxydases, Monoamino-oxydases, Diamino-oxydases, Enterokinases, Thrombokinases, Ureases.

Further substances: Cholin, Acetylcholin, Cystin, Throsin, Arginin, Histidin, Erapsin, Trypsin, Histamin, Methionin, Thromboplastin, Purnbases, Eucleoproteids, Nucleic Acid, Glycogen Iron, Calcium, Cobalt, Saturated and unsalted fatty acids.

The generally healing quality of the placenta as a whole applies to any group of its cells, and appropriate placenta cells are included in every cell injection treatment since they accentuate the effect of other glandular or organic cell injections.

Periodical injections of placenta cells are helpful in some cases. They improve the general tones and have a circulating, revitalizing, rejuvenating effect on aging systems, and upon aging skin in particular.

The skin otherwise healthy ages only through lack of circulation, and that means lack of the nourishing substances it requires. Placenta cells, by providing the increased circulation and the nourishing elements, have an effect on the skin which no external use of creams and lotions can possibly achieve.

The same thing applies to the hair. If the scalp is badly circulated the hair roots are not properly nourished and the hair becomes extra dry and brittle, breaks, falls out or turns prematurely gray. Placenta cells, with cells of the suprarenal cortex, can do much for the hair and scalp. When, however, the scalp is too tightly drawn over the skull, like a tightly fitting cap, the mechanical pressure on the blood vessels of the scalp prevents them from widening, and cell treatment cannot be effective in that region until the scalp has first been loosened by manipulation and massage. People suffering from nervous stress often have a very tight scalp.

Placenta cells are used in the following cases and conditions: after exhausting childbirth; for premature babies who tend to remain underdeveloped and underweight; in all cases of physical weakness and exhaustion, such as after a major operation; for underweight, slow-growing children; for all kinds of dysmenorrhoea; underdeveloped breasts; circulatory deficiencies such as coronary affection; swellings; oedema and chilblains; varicose veins (here repeats are often required); gastric ulcers: in ophthalmic conditions where insufficient circulation causes or aggravates the existing defect. They act as a restrictor or brake on the growth of tumors, benign or malignant, and seem to have an analgesic effect generally, which is particularly noticeable in cases of arthritis long before the actual healing process begins.

6

The Main Organs

Heart and Circulation: Heart and circulatory deficiencies, with cancer, are the chief health hazards of our time. Statistics show a forty percent rise in heart and circulatory diseases as a cause of death since the beginning of the century, with evidence of a particularly sharp uptrend after the Second World War.

Circulatory deficiencies may be caused by any condition which impedes the normal circulation of the blood through the arteries: most commonly by arteriosclerosis, which is the hardening of the arterial walls.

These two conditions nearly always occur together and, unless treated, will bring on coronary thrombosis, invalidism through hemorrhage from a burst blood vessel and, often, a stroke.

Also, since no organ is self-sufficient, arteriosclerosis is liable to be accompanied by inadequate action of other organs. This, if for instance the other organs happen to be the kidneys, may in its turn lead to renal failure or cause oedema, swellings and accumulations of fluid in various parts of the body—often visible as pouches under the eyes, puffiness of the feet, ankles and legs.

Cardiovascular disorders are largely the result of the stress and strain of modern living conditions: overdoing work and play—excesses of work are not less harmful because considered more virtuous than excesses in other directions.

The typical patient is, in fact, one who all his life has been overdoing everything: heavy responsibilities in his job, pace of work, long hours which do not leave enough time for recuperation through relaxation, rest and sleep, and result in the overburdening of the nervous system which is closely connected with circulation. This circulatory disturbance is further aggravated by regular indulgence in over-large meals which damage the fat and protein metabolism.

Add to all this the fact that coronary patients seem, unfortunately, to be oversensitive to the slightest additional strain, and that any physical, intellectual or emotional stress has a harmful effect on the circulation of the coronary area, and it is not difficult to see why the treatment of heart and circulatory complaints has become a major field of medical research in recent years.

Cell therapy can bring very satisfactory results in heart cases provided it is applied with discretion. Care is advocated for two specific reasons:

One: the patient's susceptibility to the slight additional stress in undergoing the injections.

Two: the danger which comes from the swift initial relief that is often obtained, after which patients relieved of their symptoms and feeling much better are apt to think they are strong enough to resume all their former bad habits. Nothing could be more mistaken. Repairs to a damaged heart and arteries cannot be effected in a few days. To think of these organs like a decarbonized car engine and to "step on the gas" at the first opportunity is the surest way of throwing away the good effects of treatment.

The disappearance, welcome though it is, of distressing symptoms like angina pectoris, for instance, cannot be interpreted as a complete cure. All it means is that the injected cells have "taken," and have become part of the patient and are beginning to add their quota of new vitality to his depleted organism.

In many heart cases, one or perhaps several cell treatments will achieve considerable improvement, or even a complete cure: but in chronic cases of long standing regular cell treatment at suitably spaced intervals may be needed.

Also, heart patients, like diabetics, should remain under medical supervision after treatment: a regular sensible diet must be prescribed and then kept strictly to—this will ensure an improved metabolic rate. Manipulative treatment and suitable physical exercise will also help to improve the body's general condition and efficiency.

Most important of all, medical supervision should aim at preventing all further stress for heart patients—often a baffling problem when the patient is a creative, sensitive, temperamental person in a responsible position. But tactful supervision of this kind after cell treatment is necessary in prolonging such a patient's life.

Those who have had a severe coronary deficiency before cell treatment with possibly a bad heart attack, or perhaps a stroke, will continue to remain vulnerable even after successful treatment. The duration of their lives will depend largely on the care of their physicians combined with their own cooperation. Such patients have to learn to be content with a considerably limited field of action. Again, this is not always an easy situation from either the doctor's or the patient's point of view, because this type of patient is often one who thinks he knows his limits better than his doctor.

Although the number of injections will vary with individual diagnosis, the key cells used in the treatment of sclerotic cardiac and arterial conditions, as well as in cases of cardiac and renal insufficiency and angina pectoris, are those of heart, intima (cells of the arterial walls of a fetal or very young animal), kidney, gonad and placenta.

Each has its specific action. Substantial doses of placenta cells lower the blood pressure; gonadic cells (testes for males, ovary for females) improve circulation, young intima (from the arterial walls) can make old, hardened degenerated walls of human arteries and heart elastic again, by helping to remove the cholesterol, or chalky coating, which has hardened them.

With the renewed elasticity of the arteries goes a process which improves the blood circulation in general, but especially in the brain, the heart itself and the coronary arteries.

Cells of spleen, liver and parathyroid improve the quality and consistency of the blood and effect a further reduction in the formation of cholesterol.

Cell treatment can also help even in cases of stroke, involving damage or paralysis of limbs or powers of speech; but in order to avoid additional stress it should not be given until approximately three months after the stroke has occurred. Repeat injections at intervals may ultimately produce quite astonishing results in these cases. But here once again it has to be emphasized that no results are obtainable after a severe stroke without effort on the patient's part to regain lost ability to move, walk or speak. Perseverance with re-education of affected muscles, with remedial exercises and rehabilitating occupations is absolutely essential.

The more widely known pathological heart conditions which respond to cell therapy are the following:

Damage through degenerative condition or thrombosis.

Weakness due to aging or poisoning (nicotine, alcohol, drugs).

Atrophy.

Poor development in fast-growing children.

Valve irregularities (compensated for in inducing better development of the heart muscle itself).

Sclerosis.

Cardiac asthma.

Angina pectoris.

The Lungs: When diseases of the lungs are mentioned, people tend to think immediately and only of pulmonary tuberculosis, a disease which was very prevalent a generation or two ago, but which, thanks to modern therapeutics and hygiene, is now greatly reduced in incidence.

Since tuberculosis is an infectious disease, cell therapy has not, so far, been able to effect a cure. But research into this matter is in progress.

In cases of latent tuberculosis, however, cell injections

have proved very helpful in improving the patient's general condition and in increasing his powers of resistance.

One affection of the lungs, however, which does respond well to cell therapy is asthma.

Asthma is often caused by nervous dysfunction and, like hay fever, may be an allergic condition. This type of asthma calls for treatment with lung cells, placenta and hypothalamus, the latter to improve the nervous functions. When the condition is accompanied by skin affections, such as psoriasis, the Abderhalden tests usually indicate that spleen, liver and pituitary glands are not functioning normally, and the cell therapy applied will also cover these dysfunctions.

Kidneys: The most common kidney disease, nephritis, which frequently offers resistance to chemotherapy of all kinds, responds well to cell therapy. But since dysfunctions of the kidneys often accompany various heart affections, in such cases both heart and kidneys have to be treated.

The usual cell treatment includes kidney, heart and placenta. Where, as is frequently the case, there is oedema (swelling due to retention of fluid), thyroid cells are added.

Many people are surprised to learn that eyesight and hearing can be improved by treating the kidneys. Such, however, is the case; defects of vision and hearing are often caused by renal insufficiency and soon clear up after treatment of the kidneys.

The treatment of gout through the kidneys is perhaps more obvious since gout is caused by the retention of toxic matter in the bloodstream, owing to insufficient cleansing action by the kidneys. Cell treatment for gout is therefore aimed chiefly at the kidneys and obtains good results.

Stomach, Duodenum, Intestines: Some stomachs produce insufficient gastric acid due to dysfunction of the acid-producing cells. Injection of stomach cells often clears up such dysfunctions.

Stomach cells are also indicated in cases of gastric ulcer and anemia. In the latter case they accentuate the action of injected liver and spleen cells.

Duodenum cells are helpful in cases of duodenal ulcer and deficient secretion of the gall bladder.

Liver: There is a great deal of truth in the old saying that "life depends on the liver." The organ not only plays a leading role in the processes of digestion and metabolism but also seems to be closely connected with a person's mental state.

We all know what is meant by choleric temperament, but we forget, perhaps, that the word "choleric" comes from the ancient Greek "khole," meaning bile; and that those who were considered particularly prone to anger had in fact a surfeit of "choler" or "bile" in their physical make up.

The liver is an important factory, safety valve and storage depot within the body. It is instrumental in the purification of the blood: in the unborn child, for instance, until the third month, it is the only blood-forming organ.

Bile is produced by the liver and stored within the gall bladder. Its purpose is to help break down fats to form amino acids in the metabolic process which changes food into body-building materials. If the fats are not properly broken down and chemically changed, digestive troubles ensue, varying in severity from a simple stomach upset to serious illness. All these conditions react on the mental state and temperament of the sufferer, and it is certainly true that people are not at their best when they are what is described as "liverish" or "bilious."

The liver is also the body's chief chemical laboratory.

The iron needed to produce hemoglobin, the red pigment in the blood, is stored mainly in the liver. Deficiency of hemoglobin produces a form of anemia. Many people often suffer for a lifetime from a slight or medium degree of anemia without realizing it. They never feel well; at the same time they are not really ill but constantly "under the weather," with a whole series of vague complaints.

These people can be put right by cell therapy. Injections of liver and spleen, bone marrow and, often, blood and hypothalamus cells, cause their vague and everchanging complaints to disappear.

The same cell combination in more massive doses is successful in cases of pernicious anemia.

In fact, improved liver condition usually gives a boost to the whole system. Life does indeed depend on the liver.

The following is a summary of the main conditions for which liver cells may be used in combination with other cells:

Diabetes mellitus.
Jaundice, deficient or lacking bile flow.
Cirrhosis of the liver—if not too far advanced.
Atrophy of the liver.
Pernicious anemia.
Inability to put on weight.
Convalescence after illness—to speed recovery.
States of exhaustion and debility.
Toxic states, including alcoholic and drug poisoning.
Allergies, asthma, hay fever.
Various skin affections.
Arthritis and osteoarthritis.
Varicose veins, leg ulcers, hemorrhoids.
Persistent chilblains.

The Spleen: The spleen, like the liver, is popularly associated with ill-temper: to vent one's spleen upon a person means to allow pent-up ill-will to explode in spiteful anger.

But unlike bile and the bilious, choler and the choleric, the association of ideas in the case of the spleen is obscure.

Situated on the left side just below the stomach, the spleen is a very hardworking organ, although its exact physiological function was unknown until fairly recently. Today it is considered to act as a substitute for the thymus gland which gradually fades away after puberty. Thus, while the thymus looks after the process of growth in childhood, the spleen assists in the maintenance of the body, including fighting germs, toxins and all morbid physically unhealthy tendencies, throughout adult life.

It could be called the organizer-in-chief of the whole system, keeping, as it does, a check on so many internal disorders.

It manufactures a proportion of the white corpuscles, destroys used cell components and acts as a filter for micro-organisms invading the blood stream. The lymphocites in the spleen may be compared to a demolition squad, clearing away rubbish and used building materials in the form of waste matter, impurities and toxins.

As a therapeutic agent, then, for the whole system, the spleen is closely concerned in all processes of illness and recuperation.

Treatment with spleen cells—which keep the body healthy and act as a prophylactic—is thus an important part of cell therapy.

Indeed, the prophylactic action of the spleen is regarded by some cell therapists as an illustration of the way cell therapy actually works.

The spleen contains antibodies against toxins and all invading bodies. The invading organisms are broken down into their components which are then either destroyed or neutralized or "eaten," that is to say, utilized as building components for the human system.

As foreign bodies, the injected cells are broken down into their components, useless foreign proteins are destroyed and useful materials retained to be sent, through the bloodstream, to the organ, gland or other distressed area where it is needed.

To sum up, spleen cells are included in cell injections in the following cases:

To clear the body of toxins in cases of poisoning (together with liver cells).

To promote the formation of antibodies in cases of infection (together with liver cells).

To increase the resistance to infection (together with liver cells).

To promote the healing of old wounds, festering varicose veins, etc.

To improve the condition of the blood through the introduction of additional iron, albumen, cholesterol and improving the hemoglobin level.

To desensitize allergic conditions, such as chronic asthma, hay fever, urticaria, sudden abdominal swellings, dermatitis, gastric and duodenal ulcers. To accelerate the healing process in cases of anemia.

7

The Brain

BRAIN cells do not divide and multiply in a constantly re-
curring cycle of death and renewal, as happens with other
cells; no provision exists for their complete self-renewal as
a whole entity. Considering what the brain is used for,
perhaps this is a wise dispensation—a precaution even—by
Nature. For among its other uses the brain is a storage
place for the information, images, impressions, etc., required in thought processes; so that cell renewal in the
brain would be the equivalent of renewing every printed
page and card in the catalogs and indices of a vast library
with an exceedingly complicated system of cross references. New blanks would not be much use; who wants to
begin all over again what it has already taken years to get
together and index in a certain way? To be of any help,
each new cell would have to be a photostat copy of its
predecessor, with room for further expansion; and as time
went on the renewal process would become very onerous
indeed.

Instead, then, what is replenished and renewed is the material of which the brain cells are composed, their chemical structure in fact. This process of molecular renewal is going on all the time throughout the body. In a period of six to eight months every molecule of every tissue in the body, including those of the brain, is replaced by a new one. This is important, because if the chemical structure of the brain remained constant under all conditions, very little, if anything, could be done by any therapy to remedy cerebral underdevelopment, degeneration, disease or premature senility.

Environment, stress and strain, disease and injury, including birth trauma, can and do cause considerable fluctuation and irregularity in the chemical composition of the brain, with resultant abnormalities which manifest themselves often years later. The abnormalities may be only temporary, but they tend, especially if untreated, to be permanent. Mentally retarded children, Mongols, the prematurely aged and the senile all have brains which do not function normally, though in each case from different causes. Some of these dysfunctions stem from faults in the glandular system and other physiological processes; but even when such faults are corrected, the cerebral functions often still remain subnormal or abnormal. Until quite recently it was assumed that the chemical structure of the brain was a constant, unchanging factor, so no attempt was made to reach or modify it. For mental and behavioral abnormality the only medical treatments were psychiatry, "mind" drugs and remedial training. The most positive results were achieved by the drugs, even though these had to be continued indefinitely often with undesirable side-effects. But, generally speaking, little improvement was

[76]

considered possible, and most cases were regarded as more or less hopeless.

Biological repair to the brain tissue—that is to say, repair by cell therapy—is still in the empirical stages, but research and experience show two positive results. These are the development of underdeveloped parts of the brain, and the partial or complete repair of damaged brain tissue —both as a result of the injection of brain cells.

Neither in the brain nor anywhere else does the complete cell reach its home site intact. As already explained, the chemical components of the cell—its valuable nucleic acids and ferments—reach the area where they are needed through the blood stream. By this means—that is to say, through stimulation by the injected cell material—the chemical composition of the brain cells can be normalized, so that parts underdeveloped through lack of the right chemical nutrients have a chance to develop.

The theory of molecular regeneration through the absorption of the needed components from the broken down injected cells is quite plausible and acceptable, when it is born in mind that this is also the only explanation of the process of growth of the healthy brain from birth to maturity. This being accepted, it follows that maintenance and molecular regeneration will be far better improved by the 100 percent valuable nucleic acids, hormones, vitamins and chemicals derived from injections of healthy cells than ever it could be by the same substances inferior in value by 50 percent because derived from their own degenerating, aging, diseased, declining or underdeveloped human systems. Injections of brain cells alone would, however, have little result. They are always given in conjunction with other cells prescribed in accordance with the Abderhalden test, which is able to discover exactly which areas and lobes of the brain are underfunctioning or dysfunctioning.

When cells corresponding to those areas are injected at the same time as brain cells, an improvement in various brain functions and in physical functions connected with the affected areas of the brain usually follows.

However, the number of brain cases successfully treated by cell injection is still not large enough to permit sweeping generalized claims.

The greatest amount of work in this branch of cell therapy has been done in Germany, and it is slowly developing in the United States. Apart from Professor Niehans himself, the following practitioners have reported positive results to the International Association for Cell Therapy, the president of which is Dr. H. Dahmer, a professor at Heidelberg University:

Professor Dr. H. Dyckerhoff, Cologne.

Professor Dr. H. Haubold, Munich.

Professor Dr. F. Destunis, Friedrichshain Hospital, Berlin.

Professor von Schubert, Director University Hospital, Berlin.

Professor Dr. Mommsen, Frankfurt.

Professor F. Schmit, University Clinic for Children, Heidelberg.

Profesor Dr. H. G. Rietschel, Town and Country Hospital, Herford.

Dr. Sprado, Frankfurt.

Hyman Goldstein, M.D., New York.

The most satisfactory results in this branch of cell therapy have been in cases of underdevelopment of parts of the brain, especially in the treatment of mentally and physically retarded children and Mongols. More will be said about this in the chapter on retarded children.

Much, then, has still to be learned about the brain as a physical organ. But in recent years strides have been made in research on certain parts of the brain which, because they are so closely and vitally connected with all physical and mental processes, are of major importance to the entire human system.

Today, better understanding of their concerted action makes it possible to take full advantage of the biological rebuilding processes of cell therapy; and it is significant that, whatever organ or condition is being treated by this therapy, an essential part of the diagnosis by the Abderhalden test is a check on the thalamus-hypothalamus and cerebellum for signs of under- or overfunctioning. These three organs are connected intermediaries between brain, glandular and nervous systems and unless their condition is taken into account, cell treatment may show little or no result.

The hypothalamus is the main regulator of the blood supply to the brain and has twenty-four known centers. Through these centers it is directly connected with the following functions and physiological systems: growth and formative development; the neuro-vegetative control of involuntary rhythms and movement (e.g., breathing, pulse, peristalsis, the depth and quality of the sleeping and waking state; body temperature; all endocrine functions through the pituitary gland; motor impulses (e.g., movements, posture, muscle tone); sensory reactions; metabolism; formation of the blood corpuscles and resistance power in inflammatory conditions; emotions and mental impulses with their numerous rational and physical off-shoots.

Dysfunction of the hypothalamus is very common. Its more obvious effects are shown in disturbances of sleep, recurrent severe dizziness, depressions and certain kinds of headaches. But alone or in combination with thalamus and cerebellum dysfunction, the long-term results can be disordered functioning of all organs. At first no pathological changes are discernible. A patient may complain of various aches and pains, produce all the symptoms of gastric ulcers, gallbladder trouble, various heart complaints, arthritis and other conditions, but his doctor finds nothing wrong in any of the seats of trouble. The patient is told his symptoms are functional or "nervous," and that there is nothing to worry about, since he is organically sound.

However, prolonged dysfunction of one or several organs does frequently produce pathological changes in them, and the patient then suffers from real gastric ulcers, gallbladder trouble, arthritis, heart disease, sclerosis and so on.

In the highly-strung, the nervous, neurotic and unbalanced as well as those undergoing the climacteric (premature or otherwise), and in the elderly, it can be assumed right away that the hypothalamus, thalamus and cerebellum are affected. This is confirmed in more than 90 percent of cases by the Abderhalden tests.

The hypothalamus is especially sensitive to toxins; those who have been under prolonged medical treatment, drug addicts, heavy drinkers and smokers, invariably show hypothalamic dysfunction. An immediate result of disorganization of one or more of these key junctions between the brain, the glandular and the nervous systems is some disturbance of the vegetative nervous processes which, in their turn, bring circulatory deficiency and lack of nourishing blood and nerve supply in various major organs. The harmonious concerted activity of the whole system is disrupted. Through lack of blood circulation with its supply of nourishing and building materials, more cells die than can be reproduced; a vicious circle of degeneration gathers momentum and if that circle is not somewhere decisively broken, a process of destruction continues in the various organs concerned. Additional chemotherapy—more drugs and medicines—may act as a palliative and seemingly cure the patient's symptoms. But in reality, far from helping the impaired thalamus and hypothalamus, the consumption of more drugs and medicines throws an extra burden on those organs and makes their condition worse.

In such cases, a series of cell injections, to restore the hypothalamus, the thalamus and cerebellum to a normal, healthy function, often leads to a cure of the secondary symptoms.

Approximately the same may be said about the relationship between the thalamus and the glandular system. The thalamus exerts a regulating action on the entire endocrine system, with the accent on the pituitary gland. It is therefore impossible for the glandular system, and the pituitary in particular, to function normally if the hypothalamus and, possibly its associates are out of order. Corrective treatment of the pituitary and other suspected glands may be a failure if the hypothalamus is not first investigated and, where necessary, treated.

In connection with the relationship between the hypothalamus and the glandular system, an interesting experiment has been carried out by research scientists Rosenberg and Guillamin. They noted that a pituitary culture continued to produce one of its hormones, ACTH, for three days after it had been taken from the donor. Then the culture kept on growing, but stopped producing ACTH. Two weeks later, a piece of hypothalamus was introduced into the culture without touching the original pituitary specimen. The pituitary tissue started again secreting ACTH. The experiment has been repeated and always produces the same results.

Attempts to treat damage to hypothalamus and thalamus by chemotherapy, including synthetic hormones, have not been successful. Massive doses of hormones of the pituitary and other glands are sometimes used in attempts to reach the hypothalamus and thalamus. The results are often poor and obtained at the cost of substantial damage to the glands concerned.

As the laboratory experiment described above seems to suggest, the biological approach is the right one, and practical experience corroborates this view. Injections of the corresponding cells or cell extracts are able to reach and regulate the hypothalamus and its associates. This has been proved in the treatment by cell therapy of functional and pathological conditions which did not respond to other therapeutic measures.

Certain obstinate kinds of obesity are among the conditions successfully treated. When they are caused by pituitary and hypothalamic dysfunction and do not respond to pituitary treatment alone, they have been cured by injection of glandular and hypothalamic cells. Many cases of amenorrhea, dysmenorrhea, sterility and frigidity, previously believed to be psychological and unsuccessfully treated by psychotherapy, have been cleared up by treatment containing glandular cells with the addition of hypothalamus, thalamus and cerebellum. These cells are important, too, in the treatment of all climacteric symptoms.

A particularly difficult complaint to diagnose correctly is latent mild tetany. Cramps and cramp-like conditions of any description and in any organ are, as might be expected, generally diagnosed as affections of the organ or organs concerned. Heart cramps are thought to be symptoms of heart disease or angina pectoris, colic of gallbladder or kidney is expected to be a disease of those organs, where stones are suspected as the cause. Stomach and duodenum spasms are presumed to be due to ulcers, and, to complicate matters, sometimes the patient actually *has* an ulcer.

What is remarkable in such cases of stomach or intestine spasm with ulcer is that the usual diet for ulcers does not help, and that reckless deviations from the prescribed diet are tolerated without ill consequences, as are smoking and alcohol.

The explanation is that a slight, latent tetany is the cause of the cramp symptoms, and that the organs themselves are, so far, not in a pathological condition. The same explanation goes for various cramps, spasms, shifting pains and aches all over the body, pains which invariably are diagnosed as rheumatism of some kind, osteoarthritis, neuralgia, neuritis, fibrositis, etc. The usual diagnosis of these common symptoms may often be correct, but if with the symptoms the calcium level of the blood is found to be very low, then the cause of the aches, pains and cramps is not rheumatism of any kind but a latent tetany due to a combined dysfunction of the hypothalamus and the para-thyroid glands. Only the Abderhalden diagnosis can make quite sure. The usual experience is that the cramp-like symptoms disappear with the administration of the cells of the appropriate organs after accurate diagnosis.

Hypothalamus cells are indicated in the treatment of the following conditions:

dwarfism, asymmetrical physical development, dis-orders of the nutrition-digestion-assimilation process;
hot conditions, palpitations, too-slow heart beat, "flut-terings";
spasmodic disturbance of the circulation; disturbed sleep;
disturbed secretions of sweat, tears, saliva, bile, milk, urine, juices of stomach and intestine;
imbalanced secretion of the endocrine system;
difficulties of posture and balance; dizziness;
hypotonic muscles;
insufficiency of the natural, involuntary movements of stomach and intestines;
disturbance in passing urine and feces;
disturbances in sight, hearing, taste and smell;
obesity;
two varieties of diabetes (mellitus and insipidus) if caused by the hypothalamus itself;
lack of minerals and blood formation;
disturbance in the healing process in inflammatory conditions;
various gastric, duodenal and intestinal ulcers;
disturbance of sexual potency;
depressive states and various psychological disturb-ances;
menieres syndrome.

8

Retarded Children

RETARDED children, or children showing some kind of abnormal development, account for nearly two percent of the population of Western Europe. In England and Wales alone, the estimated figure is over one million. It is therefore not surprising that the education and welfare of these children, youths and adolescents constitute a major therapeutic and social problem, the more so since statistics show their numbers are increasing, rather than the reverse.

Sociologists have shown a particular interest in the problem of the retarded and the subnormal since the First World War, when the first steep rise was recorded about 1916. The tendency towards increase has continued ever since, with another marked rise during and after the Second World War.

The causes of these unfortunate increases arise from a combination of factors more or less connected with the effects of war: abnormal stress in the first place, and the nervous and physical shocks to parents of war-time living conditions; the deferment of marriage for economic and other reasons, with the resultant higher ages of parents; lack of adequate suitable nourishment for expectant mothers—a factor more applicable to Western Europe than to Britain.

At the present time, a continuing factor seems to lie in the tendency towards a considerable disparity of age between parents. With the rise in the divorce rate goes an increase in marriages in which one of the partners—the man usually—is much older than the other. It is an established fact that, frequently, the first child of elderly parents is Mongol or Mongoloid, even though both parents may have been perfectly healthy, normal children of a previous marriage in which the ages of the parents were less unequal.

The cause of physical and mental retardation or defects in the offspring of aging parents, or even of couples of whom only one is aging, lies in the glandular and general physical conditions of the parent or parents; a condition where deficiency in the parental genes, chromosomes, hormones, etc., adds up to the inability to give the unborn child a good start in life. (This can also happen when a parent, though young in years, has prematurely aged through stress of modern life, or when premature aging may have been taking place for more than one generation).

Strangely enough, in one way, the rise in the standard of living and the more affluent society with its ever-pressing need to "keep up with the Joneses" aggravate the social problems. The stress of having to work hard for a living coupled with the desire to play hard, too, brings on premature exhaustion and other complaints of increasing complexity and severity.

The first noticeable results of the ever-growing tendency to "live it up" are that the male and female climacteric are occurring earlier and earlier in life. It follows that impotency, infertility and senility also occur more frequently and at an earlier age than previously. In other words, the whole trend is towards a lowering of biological standards, a lowering of human quality. The Welfare State and private benevolence do what they can to help the lame ducks; efforts which, though laudable from the humanitarian point of view, do not touch the root of the problem, nor do anything to stem the downward trend generation after generation.

That can be done only by a biological boost—the sort of boost which in the past was attempted by family marriage arrangements when a bid to correct the downward trend would be made through a judicious choice of marriage partners.

Today this biological boost can be given by cell therapy which attempts, through the implantation of good healthy cells, to give the child what its parents, or one of them, did not have to give. By this method congenital defects can, to some extent, be overcome and adjusted.

This is now being done even in cases of Mongol children, hitherto regarded as incurable and nonresponsive to any therapy. These unfortunate children, who used to be left to vegetate in their families or in institutions, invariably retrogressing for lack of treatment and representing a lifelong burden to relatives or the State, can now be helped. The cost of treatment is high—though most people will agree that it is justified in such cases—and results are seldom either spectacular or swift. A condition of retardation and disturbance of growth which has been there for years obviously cannot be corrected and cured in a matter of weeks or months. Biological repair—always a slow process—is extra slow in the case of Mongols or Mongoloids, and calls for a great deal of patient understanding on the part of parents, relatives and doctors.

In the normal child, the brain lobes, the glandular and nervous systems, the capacity to learn and understand, all grow slowly. In retarded children it takes longer for the underdeveloped organs first to *begin* to grow and then slowly to develop, so that considerable time often passes before any appreciable improvement is noticed.

Cell injections have to be repeated at intervals; the treatment, as it were, grows with the child over the years, each series of repeated treatments being slightly different, modified to meet the conditions of the growing child.

Even though a complete cure, that is to say, a transformation of the subnormal to the normal, is unlikely, a partial result can mean that, in later years, the patient will be able to lead a life which is to some extent useful to himself and to others. And such a partial result must also be balanced against the fact that, without treatment, the child would not have developed mentally and/or physically at all: indeed would probably have deteriorated. With these facts in mind it is possible to see that the cost of repeated treatments to achieve this partial result is still far below that of keeping for life someone who is 100 percent incapable and a burden to himself and society. These are the hard facts which have to be faced by parents and others who have the misfortune to be in charge of badly retarded children.

The earlier in life cell therapy is applied to such children, the better chance there is of improvement. Even at a later age, such as in adolescence, astonishing results are possible, and have occurred. But for patients whose retardation is congenital there is little to be done after they have reached the age of physiological maturity.

There is a marked difference between mental retardation and mental deficiency.

Mental retardation is functional; there is impaired brain function, accompanied usually by various abnormal physical and functional symptoms, but the cerebral organs are there, capable of better development.

Mental deficiency, or arrested mental development, is due to genetic influences, trauma, disease, emotional disturbances or injury to various parts of the brain. Medical diagnosis has the far from easy task of distinguishing one condition from the other in each individual patient.

Apart from the large percentage of Mongoloids and Mongols, there are those cases of schizophrenic behavior pattern, those due to prenatal development disorders, to natal brain disorders following injury or infection, or postnatal disorders of the central nervous system caused by infection. Then there are cases of brain injury, metabolic brain disorders and cerebral palsy (paralysis). Frequently children with brain disorders are born apparently quite normal; the symptoms of deterioration begin to show themselves only months or years later.

After years of trial, it is recognized today that cell therapy is the only treatment so far discovered which has any chance of achieving satisfactory or lasting results with retarded children of all types.

Professor von Schubert of Berlin, and other European

[89]

pediatric specialists, have treated countless cases of children's mental and physical retardation with cell therapy, always with some degree of success.

In general, it can be claimed that, after prolonged treatment, there is improvement in speech, intelligence, physical growth, the ability to move and coordinate movements in nearly all cases.

The cell preparations used are, as always, a matter of individual diagnosis. Usually they will include cells of the following glands and organs: pituitary, thyroid, frontal brain (for speech function), thymus (for growth), thalamus, hypothalamus, cerebellum (for all functions), cerebral cortex, cerebral marrow, other lobes of the brain, according to individual need, and always placenta to accentuate the result of treatment.

Concurrently with treatment, also for some time before and after, vitamins A, B, C, D, and E must be given. This is especially important with very young children but often their administration presents a problem because the digestive system, especially the liver, gallbladder and pancreas of physically backward children, is incapable of dealing with the vitamins from the point of view of incorporating them into the blood. The initial treatment, therefore, is aimed not at correcting the child's retardation as a whole but that of his digestive system. The slowness of the process of improvement and the reason for repeated treatments will thus be understood.

It has often been noticed that the impetus, physical and mental, given by cell treatment to the development of a retarded child tends to come to an end after approximately six to twelve months. The child's condition does not retrogress; the level of improvement, once established, remains constant, but there is no further progress until the treatment is repeated, possibly with a slightly different combination of cells.

9

Cancer Prevention

THE problem of cancer is the problem of uncontrolled cell growth through suddenly increased local division and multiplication, in rebellion against the natural pattern of cell renewal. The essence of the biological repair process is the normalizing of all bodily functions from the foundations—the cell—upwards. When functioning normally, the body has very considerable powers of resistance to disease.

Because of its ability to normalize functions, cell therapy can, according to Niehans, be looked upon as a prophylaxis against cancer whether the disease is present or not. When cancer is suspected or actually diagnosed, this prophylactic action can be used to revitalize and so strengthen glands and organs which play a leading part in the body's fight against disease.

It can stabilize a cancerous growth and prevent it from spreading, occasionally even inducing a certain amount of regression, while improving the patient's general condition to such an extent that he can carry the stabilized growth more or less as if it were a natural part of his organism.

Paul Niehans makes his claims with 40 years' experience of cell therapy and more that 42,000 recorded cases behind him, in a newly published booklet called *The Cancer Problem* (published by Stampli & Co., Berne).

In view of the fact that there is no medically accepted cure for cancer and the interest any discussion of it may arouse in a world where one person in five dies of cancer, and of the controversy which any suggestion of even a near-possible cure evokes—in view of all these considerations we have thought it best simply to reprint those parts of the booklet which provide the author, at least in his own opinion, with support for his claims.

Sometimes referring to himself as "Niehans," sometimes as "I" he writes:

Niehans considers cancer primarily as an immuno-biological problem. Cancer can be transplanted, but can also be favorably influenced in a prophylactic and therapeutic manner by injection of fetal or young revitalizing cells taken from animals with the greatest resistance, sheep for example.

The most widespread view today is still that cancer is a degeneration of aging epithelial cells, that is to say, a deficiency disease of old age which has been mastered by the cells of certain cancer-resistant animals.

There is no disease to which the body will not offer resistance. Many spontaneous cures have been recorded and described. . . . From this Niehans concluded that living creatures, both men and animals, can develop forces which inhibit or overcome even the most serious diseases, such as cancer.

Animals have inhabited our planet much longer than human beings so that it is possible that they may adapt themselves much better to their environment than human beings and have developed more resistance against disease.

For example while we know of only a few isolated cases of spontaneous cure of cancer in human beings, in the animal world there are whole species which are more or less cancer-resistant.

This marvellous fight that animals can put up against cancer, a quality acquired through millions of years of conflict against the disease, can be utilized by the human race, still lagging behind in the domain of cancer. . . .

In 1949 I experimented with implants of benign cellular cultures against malignant cellular cultures. Also I gave the first injections of fresh cells in a case of cancer of the breast; fetal spleen, fetal thymus, fetal heart muscle, fetal duodenum, fetal jejunum, placenta, ovary and epiphysis. . . .

As cancer is a matter of a generalized illness, a disturbance in the regulation of a disharmony, probably in the endocrine system—the tumor is a localized reaction at a chronically damaged spot—we must, whenever possible, carry on the war on the two fronts:

1. Against the predisposition to cancer.

This is such a formidable enemy that we must summon up against it all the forces at our disposal, *the revitalization of damaged cells* by the injection of cells taken from cancer-resistant animals.

2. Against the malignant tumor.

This can be removed by the knife when it is discovered in time. Perhaps we may soon be able to lay aside the knife (I am myself a surgeon).

Sheep are not only cancer-resistant; they are also resistant to some other diseases. As mammals they have attained a high degree of development and are found in big flocks all over the earth. It is also significant for us that they produce no poisons in their defense.

For thousands of years they have strengthened their cells in the constant fight against cancer and are victorious today.

Their cancer resistance is transmitted to man and to certain animals through cellular injections.

So that we fight with formations of millions of cells already proved in warfare against the legions of cancer cells.

Nature has provided us with sufficient militant cells. If injected in good time they are remarkably strong and prove successful.

We draw upon sheep for fetal or young cells, fresh or preserved cells, for all their cells are cancer resistant; but only those cells which the organism needs are appropriated and utilized by the human beings.

As the mature placenta contains all the nutrients that the unborn child needs for life as well as materials for defense against sickness, we use as the base of our injection for *children* mature placental cells from sheep, removed immediately before birth.

According to our statistics, probably the most comprehensive in the world, the hypothalamus (anterior, middle and posterior regions) is found damaged in almost all adult and aging patients, so for these patients we use as a base:

(1) mature placental cells, taken from cancer-resistant animals.

(2) hypothalamic cells from cancer-resistant animals. The two kinds of cells, administered separately, support one another without causing any disturbance.

Niehans has injected thousands of elderly patients with cells taken from sheep but only cells from those organs needed by the patient. In this way he was able to ensure that none of his patients came to any harm.

For women he used mainly ovarian follicular cells taken from the pregnant sheeep but without the male Berger's cells from the hilum.

Men were generally treated by ligation of the vasa afferentis testis or pure Sertoli's cells taken from virile young animals.

The questions which he sought to answer were as follows:

1. Can cancer, considered as a disease of old age, be checked by cellular revitalization?

2. Or shall we attain a cancer prophylaxis by the injection of cells from relatively cancer-resistant animals?

The second problem touched him very closely as a respected grandfather and a beloved mother died of cancer. He hoped with cells and their nutrient fluids to approach more nearly to the solution of one of the most difficult problems in medicine.

In 1928, when he had already treated more than 1,000 women suffering from difficulties due to menopause by means of ovarian follicular cells taken from sheep, he was struck by the fact that cancer rarely developed subsequently in patients who had received this treatment. That made him surmise that these cells were a protection against cancer. He has now had about 40 years of observation and the results of a questionnaire which had more than 1,000 replies. The question concerning cancer ran as follows: "As I have injected cells from cancer-resistant animals it is important for me to know if patients who conscientiously carried out my instructions have become cancer-resistant."

[96]

For comparison he put a further question to his patients: "How many of your near relatives, who have not had cellular injections, have been operated on for cancer or died of cancer?"

Among the first therapeutic results described by Niehans were these:

Ligation of the vasa afferentis testis distal at the head of the epididymis.

Gotthelf Aebischer, 69 years of age, Rue Aime-Stainlen, Vevey. (The patient allowed mention of his name). Prostatectomy, June 23, 1927, on account of prostatic carcinoma with retention of urine. The histological examination of the removed prostate in the Pathological Institute of the University of Lausanne confirmed the diagnosis.

In July 1927 X-ray irradiation. In the autumn of 1927 a return of the cancer at the site of the operation. In the scar of the skin incision a fistula was forming through which the urine flowed down continuously. Urine no longer passed through the urethra. Fever and shivering fits. On September 19, 1927, ligation of the vasa afferentis testis distal at the head of the epididymis.

By November 2, 1927 the fistula had closed up and the patient was able to pass water again without difficulty. The tumor slowly disappeared and gave rise to no further symptoms. Aebischer took up his gardener's work again.

At the end of six years the doomed man of 1927 still tarried amongst the living, criticism began to stir in medical circles. It was asserted that the recurrence of the cancer was not a malignant tumor, but merely a malignant swelling. Yet on repeated examinations the prostate was always felt as a hard tumor which, however, was no longer causing the slightest inconvenience. In

1928 I presented the patient to the surgeons' congress in Montreux.

On September 3, 1933 Aebischer died of a stroke in his 76th year. At his death the bladder was completely empty and the histological examination of the prostate, carried out again in the Pathological Institute of the University of Lausanne, showed prostatic carcinoma once more. The cancerous tumor, which had been reabsorbed after the ligation of the vasa afferentis testis distal at the head of the epididymis had remained to the end of the patient's life, six years later, without spreading.

*   *   *

Doctor, born 1883, knew that he had an inoperable cancer of the prostate and came to Clarens.

May 9, 1944 ligation of the vasa afferentis testis distal.

Every year he sent me a report, the last, dated September 16, 1947, ran as follows: "Everything is going on as well as I could wish." He is tireless at his work.

*   *   *

Cancer metastasis in the head of the femur and the pelvis. (Diagnosis made at the University of Lausanne.)

Patient, born 1888, with hip-joint trouble, became bedridden. Radiography produced a picture that three University professors interpreted as a cancerous metastasis at the head of the femur. The patient declined amputation of the leg, preferred to die. February 18, 1930. Implantation of five sheep's ovaries.

The patient is able to walk again, and now goes for long walks without getting tired. A complete cure clinically, but not anatomically and pathologically, as the tumor can still be seen in X-ray examinations.

(Period of observation: 17 years.)

*   *   *

Inoperable abdominal cancer.

Patient, born 1876, energetic, a good horsewoman, healthy until 1930 when she began to suffer from lancinating pains in the leg, and gastric troubles. An inoperable, malignant tumor with metastasis was developing.

April 8, 1930: Implantation of five sheep's ovaries.

May 20, 1930: The patient reported "I am much better."

This state of well-being continued for four-and-a-half years. Then in December 1934 the pain came back, especially in the gastric region.

January 2, 1935: Second implantation of five sheep's ovaries.

Again the patient felt extremely well, so that her doctor, a well known specialist in Paris, wrote January 4, 1937: "I must admit that the implanted glands must be extraordinarily effective to keep the patient so well up till now."

Every fresh discovery is the realization of an earlier Utopian dream. . . . Our National League for the Fight Against Cancer has informed us that 20% of the population die of cancer. But if we inject cells taken from highly cancer-resistant animals the cancer figure fell from 20% to 1.2%. That is to say, cancer-resistant animals such as sheep give mankind the strongest cancer protection hitherto known, which fact I communicated in 1966 to the Papal Academy of Sciences in Rome. . . .

*   *   *

In all humility I may now permit myself to declare that I am approaching the solution of the cancer problem.

10

The Middle Years

GENERALLY speaking, although people are living longer today, they are aging more rapidly . . . that is to say, the degenerative process which attacks the middle years is setting in earlier in life than in previous generations. Signs of premature aging can occur even at twenty. Indeed, some few years ago considerable prominence was given both by the medical and lay press to the case of a boy who was certified as have died of "old age" at seventeen.

An exception, it is true—but not unique.

In fact, of course, each individual has a different rate of wear and tear. But irrespective of age, wear and tear without replacement means aging. And durability depends on inherent capabilities and how they have been developed, on temperament and other qualities conditioned by the chemistry of the glands, and on heredity.

In all living things, especially in higher organisms like man, physical life is seen to consist first of the building up of a cell state by automatic, unremitting cell renewal and, finally, of decline and decay.

In man, as long as the short-lived cells continue to be automatically replaced by their own action throughout the body, the organism remains healthy and preserves its vitality. Decline sets in when the cells begin to falter in their ability to reproduce themselves by division. The process of decline may be slow and insidious, but the longer it continues unchecked, the more difficult it is to halt and reverse.

The German pathologist Roessle constructed a scale of organic decline and aging processes in the average human system. First he put the blood; then, in succession, the capillary system and other blood vessels, the thymus gland, the bone marrow, the lymphatic system, connective tissue, spleen, cartilage, muscles, heart, ganglia, mucous membranes of the internal organs and skin.

Unfortunately, the decline in one or a few organs and glands spreads to other systems, organs and glands, causing their premature decline through lack of nourishment or over- or underfunction. Thus the aging process gets the entire person in its grip, and this is particularly regrettable where the individual is comparatively young.

The internal and external causes of premature aging are legion but can be loosely described as "everything that has affected the individual in his life so far."

Stress and strain take many forms: years of excessively hard work will cause it in one case; years of burning the candle at both ends in another; periods of severe illness followed by inadequate recuperation; long tolerated infections, possibly first contracted in childhood; chronic septic conditions of teeth, tonsils or sinuses; faulty diet and malnutrition.

With some it can stem from misuse of drugs and medicines, especially the sedatives, tranquilizers and "pep" pills; from unwholesome living conditions, lack of physical exercise and fresh air; from strenuous amusements and "living it up"; from insufficient sleep, or the abuse of alcohol or tobacco.

Stress and strain can be caused by lack of privacy in large families; by chronic noise in towns (including permanent traffic vibrations) and in the home; by atmospheric pollution from industry and motor traffic.

Monotonous factory work can be another factor, as can rush work on conveyor belts and assembly lines; and modern phenomena such as mass meetings, mass outings, mass accommodation (the holiday camp), mass evacuation in wartime with its consequent uprooting of family life.

Many cases of premature aging originated during and after the Second World War in the stress of adjustment to post-war conditions in civil life. Many more cases originate now in the social and professional competition of "keeping up with the Joneses." Indeed, modern man has become so used to stress that he tends to accept it as a normal feature of daily life. Many people are so "in love" with their source of stress that they fail to recognize it as such and would feel thoroughly unhappy if it were removed, leaving them time to relax.

What makes stress? Anything that disturbs the biological rhythm.

Parents who work all day will soon suffer from stress if their sleep is disturbed by children crying in the night, or by youngsters returning home in the early hours without accounting for themselves. Double jobs of husbands and wives for economic reasons—so common today—can cause individual or mutual stress, showing in a whole host of ailments from indigestion and duodenal ulcers to headaches, insomnia and neurasthenia.

To all these extraneous sources must be added the possibility of internal, personal ones, such as an unhappy childhood; an unhappy marriage or problems of adolescence; lack of self-confidence; worry over personal relationships, money, children, jobs; lack of aim in life; fear of the future, of old age and illness; worry over actual or imaginary bad health; the climacteric age, with all its disturbing physical and mental conditions; or conflicts arising from difficulties in professional or social, sex or religious life.

Anybody under prolonged stress ages prematurely, and for this the doctor can offer no really constructive remedy. Obviously he cannot alter the conditions and habits of modern living. Overburdened with patients regularly presenting him with ever-changing complaints, most of which belong to the stress syndromes, all he can do is to offer some palliative which will do little more than suppress the symptoms until the patient comes back again with a different set of ailments, resulting from the same cause.

It is possible, however, through cell therapy, to treat and regenerate the stress-damaged centers in the human organism, and thus delay the aging process and enable the patient to cope better with the increased physical and mental burdens of the time.

In the aging process, premature or normal, the first and most frequent damage is to the capillary system, the network of fine blood vessels permeating the whole body and supplying materials via the blood to the parts of the body involved in metabolism and assimilation (part of which is the conversion of food, water and oxygen into protein for building and repair purposes).

The outward signs of such damage are constant tiredness, sheer exhaustion, weakness, lack of energy and vitality, depression, dizziness, indigestion, insomnia, constipation, rheumatism, lumbago, etc.—a whole picture of ever-changing symptoms know as general debility.

The condition of general debility is often a result of dysfunction of liver, suprarenal glands and cerebellum, and responds well to cell therapy.

Appropriate treatment consists of substantial doses of the cells of the dysfunctioning glands and organs, plus gonadic cells, placenta and others given in general treatment of the middle-aged—although, of course, general debility can occur at any age.

Backache, often wrongly diagnosed as rheumatic but really due to degenerative processes in the spine, is another clear indication for the use of cell therapy in middle age.

Insufficiency of heart action and the circulatory system with all their attendant implications, like premature decline of sexual potency, cerebral sclerosis and arteriosclerosis, are also conditions associated with the middle years which respond well to injections of the appropriate cells.

When no pathological condition can be discovered in any organ, there is often a tendency to treat the symptoms— tiredness, insomnia, irritability, neurasthenia—lightly. This is wrong. Such symptoms arise from disturbed functioning of the vegetative nervous system and the circulatory system; if neglected they give rise to complex destructive organic processes in the entire human organism.

[104]

The combined action of the nervous and glandular systems extends into all layers and regions of the body, mind and personality. Changes in the function and structure of this system are liable to alter a person completely or change him prematurely. The stress of prolonged chronic dysfunction is a formative factor in organic disease. The first signs are a lessening of resistance and immunity to infections and disease.

Also inherent to the middle years are a whole series of complaints, now loosely grouped under the heading "manager syndrome" because they occur most frequently in those who work hard and hold responsible positions. They are due to stress; they cause excessive wear and tear, and add up to premature aging.

These symptoms can be grouped under two headings; subjective and objective. Typical of the first, the subjective, are:

Unbalanced mental states, moodiness, temporary or chronic depression, hypochondria, hysteria, restlessness, unfounded fears, listlessness and loss of initiative; tendency to isolation, masturbation, nervous and mental hypersensitivity; slowing down of reaction time; difficulty in concentration; lack of memory; the urge to rest without being able to relax, sleep disturbance and abnormally light sleep, waking tired in the morning; frequent nightmares which can be nerve-racking; general heaviness of the entire body and extremities; dizziness; chronic or frequent headache and migraine; cold hands and feet, or general feelings of cold; inability to tolerate changes in temperature and exposure to sunshine; oversensitivity to atmospheric pressure change of full moon phase; oversensitivity to pain or changes in diet; indigestion, constipation and erratic appetite; nausea; "butterflies in the stomach"; sudden perspirations and palpitations after the slightest extra physical or mental exertion; frequency of urinating; various kinds of sexual disturbances; frigidity, amenorrhea.

Objective symptoms of the "manager syndrome" include:

Frequent changes of body weight; skin troubles, blotches, rashes, urticaries; tremor of hands and body; frequent changes in body temperature and blood pressure, which may be generally too high or too low; changes in the composition of the blood; anemia; some form of diabetes; visual disturbances; changes in the hormone production of several glands; falling hair, brittle nails, various gastric disturbances.

Even though the patient may be complaining of several, or many, of these symptoms, it may well be that, at the time he decides tentatively to have them investigated, there is nothing much organically wrong.

The pity is that he often has to wait until there *is* something organically wrong before his general practitioner takes much notice of him. In this first instance he is more likely than not to be told that it is all "just nerves," to be given a tonic, tranquilizers or "pep" pills and advised to take a holiday—not much use in the circumstances since he would take his unrest, his stress and all his other symptoms along with him.

But the Abderhalden test which precedes all cell injections would almost certainly show, in cases of this kind, a dysfunction of various organs and glands and, above all, a derangement of the thalamus, hypothalamus, cerebellum or parathyroids.

These organs, singly or combined, control an extensive

series of physical, nervous and mental functions and are closely connected with the kind of disorders mentioned above.

If the dysfunctions are corrected in time, worse can be prevented and the patient given a chance to recover before his condition deteriorates until it becomes chronic and he ends up old and senile long before his time.

A critical period for the middle-aged of both sexes is the climacteric, or "change of life."

Although this is usually believed to be a female problem only, connected with the cessation of menstruation, it is a fact that men also undergo a change of life—the climacteric virile. This is less clearly marked than that of a woman but is also accompanied by physical and mental changes and difficulties.

The female menopause is often a stormy period, with conspicuous changes in a woman's physical system, state of health, nervous condition and entire personality.

The male climacteric, due to impaired testicular function, is less noticeable but often stretches over a far longer period.

Apart from the well-known hot flushes and sudden perspirations which are peculiar to the female climacteric, symptoms are more or less the same in both sexes: circulatory disturbances with headaches, loss of vitality and energy, physical decline, irritability, unreasonableness, depression and moodiness.

Injections of placenta cells have a marked effect in improving the circulatory deficiencies, while at the same time relieving a great many vague complaints, from lack of staying power and intermittent or permanent lack of powers of concentration and memory to hot flushes and excessive perspiration.

Additional injections of ovary or testes cells can, according to dosage, achieve a revitalization of the entire system, including libido and potency. In female patients the menstrual function can be revived. This is not always wished, however, by the patient and the matter should be discussed in advance so that the dosage of gonad cells can be regulated accordingly.

When in addition to the physical condition the patient has acute psychological symptoms—depression, mental imbalance and various nervous complaints—this indicates a dysfunction of the thalamus, hypothalamus and cerebellum. Appropriate cell injections will then be included in the treatment.

Climacteric disorders are among the easiest to put right by cell therapy. There is a revitalization of the entire personality, an increase in mental activity and brain function, in alertness and efficiency.

The appearance, too, is improved, owing among other things to better circulation and the effects of placenta and gonad cells on skin and hair.

It would be foolish to claim "rejuvenation": men and women in their fifties do not look twenty-five overnight. The result is more subtle: to their friends they "look good" and seem suddenly more vital and interesting, whereas before even friendly reports found them "gone off a lot" and "listless and edgy."

11

Old Age

As pointed out in the last chapter, each new population census reveals that more people are staying alive longer, slowly pushing upwards the average age of mortality.

The expected life span today of people born in Britain is 73 for females and 68 for males—as high as anywhere in the world except Norway, Denmark, the Netherlands and the United States, where they improve on these figures by a year or two. At the beginning of the century, 48 to 50 was the average length of life in Britain, and two centuries ago is was as low as 35.

But what about the quality of these lengthened lives? A look beneath the surface of the statistics reveals that many of them belong to chronic, helpless invalids and to people so handicapped mentally and physically that they constitute a major problem in the welfare state. In a comparatively short time, this problem has led to the development of a thriving new department of clinical medicine: geriatrics, the medical care of the aged, based on gerontology, the science of the processes of aging after the peak of maturity has been reached.

Unfortunately, however, the thriving is more in the practice of geriatric medicine than in those practiced upon—the husks and decrepit relics for whose benefits, in theory, the medical welfare machine for the aged exists.

It is true that old people are being kept alive—but only barely. The quality of their living may be assessed in any geriatric welfare home or hospital unit; in most cases it is that of a vegetable.

It is sad to see a human being reduced to the living capacity of a vegetable, a process, of course, which has been slowly going on over the years and for which geriatric practice is in no way responsible.

And it is disquieting to notice that this pathetic degradation is more or less taken for granted, because this infers a lowering of standards in what is generally expected from life as the years go by. It also suggests more than a hint of cynicism in its ever-growing provision of homes where the old folk may be put out of the way, burdens to no one but the professional paid to look after them.

For many of these old people, geriatric treatment amounts to being put into and taken out of their chairs day after day like so many sacks of flour, led here and there, washed and dressed, fed and finally tucked up in bed; in other words being kept physically as comfortable and as clean as possible.

This is excellent, so far as it goes. A person reduced to the level of a vegetable is far better off vegetating in an organized hygienic manner than left to do so in helpless decay, want and squalor. The crucial question, however, is: how many of these human beings *need* be so reduced? Even inherent limitations can be partly reversed and normalized, if dealt with in time.

Here, in the fields of gerontology and geriatrics, cell injections offer the widest possible scope for the necessary biological repair, revitalization and regeneration, offering the prospect of a longer life which is not just a twilight half-life bereft of the physical and mental capacity to make use of the added years.

At the lowest estimate, the elderly should be able to take life in through the five senses and be reasonably mobile on the feet and reasonably alert in the mind.

Perhaps we should emphasize here that the term "elderly" these days does not necessarily apply to people in their eighties and nineties; the growing phenomenon of premature aging sees to that. "Elderly" must be used to refer to any age after growth has ceased.

That far too many people who die well within the present life span have ceased to live long before their actual death is due to the pressure and pace of modern living which are such that, no sooner has growth ceased than a process of premature aging often sets in. The case referred to in the last chapter of the boy of seventeen who died of old age— with a degree of degeneration of organs, tissues, arteries and glands usually encountered only in an unhealthy octogenarian—is, as we said, rare but not unique. Slow premature aging begins in the average person today from the thirtieth year and, as already pointed out, may even have begun before birth!

We have already seen how it is that many modern children are "born old," the offspring of parents themselves so debilitated physically and mentally that the children simply did not get enough life force at the time of their conception. They were deprived, as it were, on their way into life, their glandular functions below par, or out of balance, their mental and physical development retarded, their whole metabolism abnormal.

Never robust, such people are ill-equipped to meet the stress of modern life, and their slender store of vitality declines at an abnormally early age. The worst cases, as we have seen, are congenitally so deprived that they are Mongols, or to some degree, Mongoloid.

People still use the expression "venerable grey beards" as a synonym for wisdom, knowledge and understanding of the kind that only long experience of a well-used life can bring. But there are few such left in sophisticated society today. The disappearance of these figures—the patriarchs (or matriarchs) who ruled benignly over a numerous household of four or five generations—and the changed social customs affecting family and tribal unity cannot, however, diminish the truth of their image. Added to the right basic material, age and experience *do* bring wisdom. Society is the poorer today for the comparative absence of the fruits of experience—contentment, serenity, sound judgment. But these are not qualities which come with premature aging, however clever the prematurely aged may be.

The "rat race" of social and economic competition is inconsistent with growing old gracefully, but is highly conducive to, say, hardening of the arteries and other symptoms of premature aging. Today the physical condition of many people in their fifties is appropriate to people several decades older, and when it comes to mental stamina and powers of concentration, the degree of deterioration can be even worse—all the more deplorable in this latter instance because, contrary to general belief, the *natural* rate of mental decline with age is very low.

Psychological tests demonstrate, for instance, that learning ability at the age of eight is approximately the same as at twelve, the peak age for learning being 22. The decline then, spread as it is over sixty years—22 to 80—is a slow process compared with the rapid ten-year development period from 12 to 22; and learning ability is only one exercise of a well-cultivated mind.

The trouble is that we are now so conditioned to premature senescence and decrepitude that age alone is a disqualification in most business and professional appointments. Youth and ineptitude are preferred to maturity and proven experience; the middle-aged are distrusted almost universally no matter how good their record is and no matter how capable they may be.

Aging is a natural process, a cosmic law; there is no point in trying to reverse it. But the physiological and mental processes of aging can be slowed down, and *premature aging,* the scourge of our times, reversed to a point normal and natural to the individual.

This means a tremendous improvement in active living quality. The middle-aged and elderly, suffering from physical and mental decline, disease and degeneration, can be made to feel years younger, so that they act and look as if they were different, healthier, happier people. In the very old and senile, spectacular changes cannot reasonably be expected; but even there the patient can be revitalized and rehabilitated to such a degree that he is no longer lifeless, useless and a burden to himself and others. That in itself can seem spectacular enough, constituting as it does a change from passive vegetation to at least some degree of active participation in life.

From the physiological point of view, aging must be looked at as a disease which, in the case of modern man as we have shown, often starts prematurely. It is believed that in an aging person, individual cells densify and shrink, the shrinkage being due to a decline in the function of the sex glands, or gonads.

The internal secretions of the gonads account for the blossoming of the young organism at puberty. Thus aging may be compared to a slow process of castration, and castration shortens life. It is a matter of common observation that a stallion lives longer than a gelding, a tomcat longer than a cat which has been neutered.

In the practice of cellular therapy, then, the key to the treatment of premature aging and all the resultant conditions of degeneration and decline is in the sex glands. There is enough life concentrated in the secretions of the male and female gonads to be the source of thousands of new living beings. It is not therefore surprising that the introduction of gonad cells is the most powerful agent in the restoration of failing vital force. A man ages when the action of his sertoli cells declines; the formation of spermatozoa stops and, for the lack of various hormones, the entire body gradually shrinks and declines. Decline, as we have seen, is a process of cells dying on a large scale without replacement, or the production of mutated cells.

The standard, nonspecific cell treatment for elderly men, therefore, always includes injection of testes cells, even though patients may be far beyond the age of sexual activity.

Similarly, the standard, nonspecific cell treatment for

aging female patients includes injection of ovary cells. A woman begins to age at the climacteric when the corpus luteum no longer does its monthly duty, circulating the entire system periodically with its hormones.

Next in importance in the process of aging are the decline of the thyroid gland, then of the central nervous system, the hypothalamus, thalamus and cerebellum.

Like the gonads, an old thyroid shrinks with the years from a normal approximate weight of one ounce to one-third of an ounce; and structural and functional changes in the central nervous system are instrumental in precipitating the aging process, causing a gradually increasing atrophy in all organs.

Results of the Abderhalden tests nearly always show an underfunction of the hypothalamus with its twenty-four separate functional centers, the thalamus and the cerebellum. Cells of one or more of these organs are nearly always included in the general biological repair treatment of the aging.

The pity is that people so often wait until they are really old and very much on the decline before they think about having treatment. Then, in sudden panic, they want to buy back life. They are ill and full of complaints, which their doctors seem to find no means of curing, but they still want to go on living and be given hope. Often these people come for regenerative therapy twenty years too late; and they have to be told not to expect miracles.

One of the main aims and possibilities of cell therapy is precisely the *avoidance* of ailing old age. If resorted to in time, it can bestow the physical and mental means of enjoying an active, healthy and happy time in the later years of life.

12

Reaction and
Follow-up

IN assessing the true value of cell therapy, it is necessary to draw a distinction between the permanent or long-lasting effects, and the temporary effects of treatment.

Permanent effects are not immediately noticeable. As we have seen, cell injections do not produce an "overnight miracle" of rejuvenation. The overall reaction is slow, often very slow. However, it is a rule of nature that what develops slowly is long-lasting; and the biological repair process of cell therapy is no exception.

The chief temporary effects are, on the credit side, a certain feeling of euphoria, causing the patient to imagine that all his ills have vanished within a few days of injection; and an immediate positive reaction—but it must be stressed a very temporary one—to the injection of glandular cells containing hormones. On the debit side there can be a fleeting recurrence of the patient's previous illnesses, even childhood ones; and, occasionally, a certain soreness for a few days at the site of the injections, the buttocks.

Serious stress reactions are very rare indeed. Where the practitioner who is giving the treatment foresees any possibility of their occurrence, he has an alternative type of cell preparation at his disposal. This is a cell extract instead of the whole cell. In the extract, the protein in the cell nucleus—which is the element believed to be responsible for the discomfort and stress sensations in cases of extreme weakness, great age and personal idiosyncrasy—is left out.

In all cases, however, the impact of cell injection does produce a *slight* degree of stress reaction. For this reason, following injection, patients are ordered to stay in bed for three days and, thereafter, to abstain from strenuous activity for three or four weeks.

When, for some reason, it is desirable to eliminate even this slight normal amount of reaction—it may be that the patient cannot afford the time to stay in bed and take things quietly; it may be that age, illness, general condition or allergic tendencies make it imperative to spare him any further strain whatever—in all such cases, instead of whole cell, the aforementioned extracts omitting the protein are used. These cell extracts are easily tolerated even by the gravely ill, the allergic and infants under one year old.

Extracts may also be used as an introduction to the full cell treatment. This is particularly useful where patients are greatly debilitated. The extract injections can strengthen them to the point where they are fit to tolerate the full treatment.

Again, extracts may be used where a quick result is wanted, since they do have a more rapid effect than the whole cell treatment; but it has to be pointed out that these effects will be of shorter duration, and will require follow-up treatment which can become very expensive.

The disadvantages attendant upon treatment with whole cells are overcome easily: the stress reaction which, in cases of substantial cell treatment to weakened patients, may take the form of a feeling of oncoming illness, and may last several days, is of little consequence: the patient deals with it by carrying out his instructions to stay in bed and rest.

The feeling of euphoria, which sometimes occurs between two and five days after cell treatment, is caused by the newly introduced RNA, which at once halts further deterioration in the organs being treated. The patient's own cells are being activated, and this produces an apparent quick improvement in the organs under treatment, and in his own general condition. But it is a very fleeting phase, and not to be trusted. The patient has to be warned that his sudden feeling of well-being will not last and that before he feels permanently better he will return to the state he was in before injection. The injected RNA *is* increasing daily and new cells *are* being formed, but it all takes time.

The injection of some glandular cells, especially those of the suprarenals, also induces a quick positive reaction which is only of short duration. This immediate, but very temporary, reaction is caused by a certain amount of hormone, or adrenaline, for instance, which is present in the injected cells.

Sometimes too, shortly after injections, former illnesses and disorders recur acutely in quick succession in reverse order, back to childhood, each lasting usually only a matter of minutes. There is no explanation for these reactions, but they need not cause alarm.

Finally, patients with allergic tendencies who react to the injections with a rash are given antihistamine, and the condition soon clears up.

The first signs of long-term improvement after cell injections vary with the patient: they may begin to be felt within four to eight weeks; they may take as long as from seven to eight months. Each individual reacts differently according to his own psychological time.

Some glandular cells show a first effect after four to six weeks. Hypothalamus cells may begin to work after eight weeks. Nerve and brain cells take longer.

If organic degeneration and destruction are advanced and the patient's general condition is very poor, or if he is very old, the process of regeneration is correspondingly slow. In a few such cases a whole year has sometimes passed without sign of improvement. One of these slow to react was an elderly woman who had been in and out of hospital for thirty-five years. She had a complicated cell treatment in December of one year; and then for a long time her condition was far worse than before. Only in the following July, seven months after treatment, did she begin to react positively. Later she recovered completely.

It sometimes happens that a first cell treatment shows no reaction whatever. In such cases a second attempt should be made, three to six months after the first. Such repeats are seldom necessary, but when given they usually show the desired result.

Patients who do not react at all are few. But where results continue to be slight, a booster injection may be given, or the treatment continued with cell extracts. If there is insufficient result on one or two counts only, the cells which show the least result may be repeated as before, or in extract form. For example, when the general result of a cell treatment is satisfactory but blood pressure or heart show little improvement, cells of heart, placenta and perhaps hypothalamus may be repeated—several times, if necessary.

Again, supposing a male patient's general condition improves after cell treatment but he still remains impotent, gonad cell injections may be repeated monthly, bi-monthly, or as the case requires.

In another case, say that of a female patient whose skin, after cell treatment, remains in a bad condition, despite an otherwise good all-round improvement, a certain number of repeat injections of placenta, with perhaps other cells, are indicated.

Cell treatment, given to restore normal health after a single acute illness, is usually permanent in its effects with no repeat needed for that particular condition.

Cell treatments given for generalized degenerative conditions should, in general, be repeated after a lapse of several years, when the patient shows signs of sliding back to the condition he was in before the first treatment. His second treatment, more often than not, has to include more cell preparations because he has aged in the meantime, or because some additional dysfunction is diagnosed. And it has to be born in mind that no medical science, no power on earth, can in the long run win the fight against time. Sooner or later old age must come on; what can be avoided is old age synonymous with ill-health and mental deterioration.

Vague stories told about the dangers of cell injections may be discounted or ignored; currently, they are without justification. It is true that many years ago, when cellular therapy was in its infancy and its practice still rare and virtually unknown, it sometimes happened that insufficiently sterilized, toxic preparations were administered, and, quite understandably, the patient did not react well.

Niehans himself, in his deliberate self-experiments in 1949, is a case in point. As related earlier, he nearly died after injecting himself with a frozen cell preparation which had become toxic. But during the past 40 years he claims that he has carried out more than 42,000 injections without a single fatality.

In any case, for many years now the cell preparations are treated and processed in state-controlled laboratories supervised by biologists and pharmacologists. There have not been, and neither can there be, further incidents from the administration of toxic preparations, of the kind that so nearly killed Niehans.

The worst that can happen to a patient is that the treatment may have no effect. But this is rare when the practitioner is a skilled diagnostician and cell therapist. Such a practitioner can judge the right amounts of the correct cell preparations to administer, and the treatment then, usually, is successful.

The importance of the role played by the practitioner in the successful administration of cell therapy cannot be overstated.

For example, underfunction of a gland can be corrected by injection of the cells of the corresponding gland, with the result that normal physiological function is resumed. If, however, a dysfunction of some kind is diagnosed, without discovering whether the dysfunction is sub- or overnormal, wrongly applied glandular cell treatment could be harmful. It goes without saying that, if an already overfunctioning gland or part of it is further stimulated by cell injections, the result will be increased overfunction, accentuated pathological symptoms and further deterioration of the patient's condition.

Or, to take another typical example, where there is an imbalance of the thyroid and parathyroid glands, the over- or underfunctioning results in a series of opposite symptoms, and it is absolutely essential that diagnosis and treatment be completely accurate.

The same principle applies in cases of pituitary dysfunction. The pituitary gland secretes twenty-four known hormones. Very often, though not always, this gland, or its anterior part, is in a state of hyperfunction when middle age is reached. If this gland, which is considered the master key to the whole glandular system, is further stimulated, partly or wholly, the entire system may be put out of gear.

That, at least, is the case in theory; in practice less harm seems to be done than might be expected; and many practitioners maintain that stimulation of a partly overactive pituitary gland balances itself out, and that the ultimate benefit of an increased output of failing hormones outweighs the temporary change.

Perhaps we should recall here the fact that Niehans regards the administration of unwanted cells as quite harmless, since the body uses what it needs and eliminates the rest, and points out that this view does not apply to cell injections for glandular deficiency. If a gland is overfunctioning, it should not be directly treated with cells at all but its antagonists stimulated with suitable cell injections so that, in this way, the hyperfunction of the first gland is reduced and corrected. In cases, for instance, of an overfunctioning pituitary gland, cells of the target glands are administered and the overproduction of the pituitary is thus counteracted.

Endocrine irregularities seldom occur singly: most glandular disturbance is pluri-glandular. Treatment has to consist of injection of cells of several glands and of cells of several organs affected by the glandular dysfunction. If treatment of the diseased organs is neglected, their condition throws such a burden on the slowly recovering and regenerating glands that they do not have sufficient chance to regain fully their normal functioning.

It is of the utmost importance, therefore, that all cell treatments be given by an experienced practitioner with a deep knowledge of his subject and everything that it involves.

13

Stress —
The Scourge of
Our Times

IN recent years stress has become a major subject of medical research in its own right. One world authority—Dr. Hans Salye of the Institute of Experimental Medicine and Surgery at Montreal University—goes so far as to say he believes almost all disease, under whatever name, is a manifestation of stress, that is to say, a result of chemical imbalance in the body caused by stress.

It is a term, too, which by now will be quite familiar to readers of this book. But familiarity is not always the same thing as understanding, and some people may still find their ideas of stress, and stress complaints and conditions, a little vague.

A good simple definition is: *Stress is the physical or mental effect of disturbance of, or interference with, any of the body's automatic biological processes.*

These processes all serve two inseparable basic wants: the maintenance of the chemical balance, and the mole-

[124]

cular and cellular renewal by which the body's *status quo* —good, bad or indifferent—is kept up. It is a self regenerating system: but not a self-sufficient and independent one. It is in fact far more vulnerable to extraneous influences than most people realize.

Extraneous influences can and do disturb automatic biological processes. Each time such a disturbance happens—and it may be a dozen times a day—it is the equivalent of throwing a wrench into the physiological works.

Take the heart, which goes on and on pumping the blood through the arteries from the moment of birth to the moment of death.

A tremendous, totally unexpected bang near at hand is within the experience of most people . . . a crashed aircraft exploding, or merely a burst tire. . . . What does it do to the automatic action of the heart?

The somersaults, pounding, thudding, racing, and other signs of disturbed heart action are accompanied by simultaneous disturbances in every cell in the body. The signals for danger are up everywhere. The first of them come quicker than any lightning flash from the sensory nerves. The glands, notably the pituitary under the brain and the suprarenals on top of the kidneys, work frantically, pouring out extra supplies of hormones into the blood stream.

These two glands have many duties, one of the chief of them being the adaptation of the organism to stress. By their increased hormone production, they counteract any threat to physical well-being. When we feel cold, their hormones constrict the capillaries and reduce peripheral circulation, thereby preserving body heat. When we are cut or wounded, their hormones increase resistance to infection, reduce hemorrhage by vasor-constriction, and reduce the blood sugar level by increasing its intake by muscle cells to provide energy.

In the case of a potentially dangerous situation, like the sudden shock of an unexpected bang, the secretion of extra hormones by these two glands prepares the body for self-defense. And, for the time being, chemical balance within the body is profoundly disturbed.

The body, however, struggles on as best it can, always seeking to return to normal by adjusting and accommodating its sensitive, finely-tuned mechanism. But it is uphill work—in fact, STRESS.

The beginning of stress is tension. We tense our muscles for action and relax them when the action is over. Tension followed by relaxation, even if constantly repeated, is not injurious. It is a natural process; it happens every time we inhale and exhale deeply. *Stress* begins when the tension is sustained with no adequate outlet in action.

For instance, suppose there has been some great disaster —an earthquake, a mining accident, or a big train crash. People who are worrying about the fate of friends or relatives involved in it are undergoing various degrees of mental and emotional stress and strain which are having definite effects on their physical organism. *Their* stress is far less healthy than that of the rescue workers, doctors, nurses, etc., even though these people may be driving themselves to the point of exhaustion in their efforts to save life. It is less healthy because it involves frustration. The energy released by the extra hormones poured into the blood—Nature's automatic response to the mental-emotional stimulus—has no outlet beyond pacing up and down, chain-smoking, incessant talking, telephoning, and useless movement.

[126]

Disasters, large and small, happen in life all the time, and we should be less than human if we did not react to them emotionally. Nevertheless, despite the physical wear and tear they inflict on us, our glands and their dependencies will not let us down for a long time, provided there is a sufficient recovery period after each onset of stress.

But this recovery period, or break in the tension, is just what we do not get today. Not only are the pressures of modern life constantly increasing, but on top of that we subject ourselves to other forms of stress, often of our own making.

Whatever capacity for serenity and relaxation we once had we now seem to have lost. We worry and hurry all day long and, even in our artificially induced sleep at night, we do not relax.

Tension, then, for whole sections of people, continues day and night. They wake up in the morning feeling jaded, unfit for work, afraid of facing the new day. They resort once again to pep pills, coffee and cigarettes or tranquilizers, and so the vicious circle goes on.

The shocks, tensions, anxieties, bad habits, mass follies and general toxic conditions of daily life add up to a prolonged accumulation of stresses. Big worries combine with little ones to make an assault on the nervous system. The automatic response of the various glands is to pour increased supplies of hormones into the blood, while their partners, or antagonists, are goaded into action to maintain some sort of working balance with the extra hormones.

Whether the worries are real or imaginary, in terms of physical damage the results are the same. Stress complaints fill the doctors' waiting rooms. In London alone, some four million persons are regularly on the doctors' lists. Beneath their various symptoms is one common denominator: anxiety—anxiety about the future, about ill-health (which, of course, only makes it worse), about all sorts of tangible and intangible problems, even about death.

In such anxiety states, there is no let up, respite or escape from tension; the worry habit has become a chronic condition. So that, as already pointed out, doctors all tell the same tale: 80 percent of all illness is caused by stress and tension of some kind; the remaining 20 percent is aggravated by stress and tension.

The doctor in the wealthier sections of the city may see more cases of high blood pressure, gastric ulcers, arterial hardening and heart trouble; the doctor in the poorer sections, more rheumatism, arthritis and circulatory diseases. But basically there is no difference: stress has its victims everywhere.

Numbers of successful business executives hold down their jobs at the cost of never-ending anxiety and tension. It is not unusual for a dignified and apparently well-controlled patient to burst into tears in the doctor's consulting room. (If he had done this more often he might never have reached the pitch of tension, and his physical condition would have been better as well.) And no matter what his physical complaint, at its roots will lie the prolonged tension of anxiety, which has strained his body's adjustment mechanism to the point of exhaustion.

Differences in constitution and heredity account for the various forms the complaint takes, which are probably at first diagnosed by the overworked doctor as functional; and he is probably so used to them that he does not take them too seriously. But if such comparatively slight functional disorders were taken in hand at the time, worse could often be avoided. It is the long-term effect of continuous stress that finally does the damage, serious damage which results in a fatal stroke, or in thrombosis and incapacity for the rest of a shortened life.

Disease, as we have repeatedly pointed out, develops in the cells, imperceptible to all conventional diagnostic methods. But the exact condition of these cells *can be* ascertained by the Abderhalden tests on which cell therapy is based. The pity is that there are only three laboratories in the world where these tests can be carried out. They should be, and no doubt one day will become, a routine part of all clinical examination, like blood pressure measurement and temperature taking.

The chief producers of stress, then, are worry, anxiety and unhappiness: mental states, it is true, but giving rise to very definite conditions.

Dr. Kenneth Appel, at one time president of the United States Commission on Mental Illness and Health, goes so far as to say that unhappiness may be the principal cause of death in modern society. He, too, attributes the enormous increase in coronary thrombosis, strokes, ulcers and high blood pressure to ever-increasing tension. And it does seem evident that, in the long run, satisfaction of basic needs is as important as nutrition in the preservation of health. Frustration of basic needs produces tension; frustrated people are not happy. If tensions become overwhelming they produce dangerous or fatal illnesses.

In the same way, those who are chronically ill, the incurable, the physically handicapped or deformed, often develop a "nasty mind," a sadistic streak or a mental imbalance which can lead to insanity or suicide. All of which emphasizes the close relationship between psychosomatic illness, which is physical illness produced by prolonged mental and emotional stress, and somatopsychic illness, which is mental imbalance resulting from prolonged physical strain and tension.

Emotional stress in pregnancy can, in some cases, lead to damage in some form to the child. For example, a mother-to-be discovers a history of mental or physical abnormality in the family, and her fear and anxiety that her child may not be normal can actually act as a magnet attracting the very condition she feared, whereas other children born before she had heard about the family "skeleton" were normal.

On the physical count, it is well-known that German measles in the first three months of pregnancy can have a catastrophic or even a fatal effect on the unborn child.

Apart from these (or similar) external physical or emotional stresses, there are various mysterious internal ones brought on by pregnancy itself, such as continual bleeding, nervous tension and toxemia. The latter is a little understood and badly defined condition, possibly caused by unidentified poisons, which is accompanied by high blood pressure and liver and kidney complaints. The unborn child can be affected. If he escapes its more serious consequences—deformity, mental or physical retardation, or some form of anemia, for instance—he is fortunate. But, at best, he is likely to be sickly and delicate, and in such cases both infant and maternal mortality are extremely high.

The effect of mental stress on the human heart, and its relation to the clogging of the arteries with cholesterol, is still a baffling puzzle. It is known that cholesterol, a fatty substance which may be forced into the walls of the arteries, can make them narrower and harden them. Too much animal fat in the diet is believed to be responsible for a high cholesterol level and arterial hardening—for arteriosclerosis in fact. Yet there are countless people who eat large amounts of animal fat in the form of cream, milk, butter, etc., without ever contracting arteriosclerosis. Their cholesterol is carried evenly with the blood through the body and their arterial walls show little or no hardening.

After nearly twenty years' research, a small group of scientists led by Dr. T. Blumenthal, laboratory director of a hospital in St. Louis in the United States, have come to the conclusion that the main cause of arteriosclerosis is not to be found in the diet but in *stress*. The cholesterol may be there, but it requires stress to make is dangerous.

Here it seems that emotional stress is the worse kind. It has been proved that emotions have a measurable effect on the cholesterol level of the blood, causing it to rise and sink.

The Medical Research Foundation of Oklahoma has published reports of tests made on patients. One man's cholesterol level reached its peak when another patient called him names and wanted to start a fight. Another patient's cholesterol level depended upon the temper of his wife. A woman patient was given another doctor when it was found that the first one always increased her cholesterol level—she simply did not like him. During pleasant interviews, patients' cholesterol level remained stable, but when deep-rooted problems were touched on, it shot up.

The study of blood flow and pressure within the arterial walls has thus led scientists to the conclusion that it is not so much the presence of cholesterol in the blood stream, as constantly fluctuating pressure and turbulence of flow that causes the arterial hardening and lesions. Coating and hardening of the arterial walls is not the same everywhere. Under the influence of stress, the two processes tend to be concentrated at arterial junctions which, because they no longer contract and expand easily with changing blood pressure, become the danger points in the arterial system. It is therefore true that a high cholesterol level is, on the whole, more conducive to arterial hardening than a low one, but it needs the stimulus of stress to become dangerous.

Given, then, this high cholesterol level, combined with emotional or physical stress and consequent unstable blood pressure, it becomes clear that the main cause of arterio-sclerosis, heart attacks, strokes and hemorrhages is stress.

Scientific experiments are not needed to show that stress is at the root of the various digestive troubles which are also constantly increasing. The nature and quality of the food eaten has little or nothing to do with them. Nervous tension, suppressed feelings of aggression or frustration, can play far greater havoc with the digestive system than, for instance, eating meals in a hurry. Nervous tension of some sort during meals can and does cause duodenal ulcers. The highest incidence is among the professional classes. Doctors, lawyers, business executives are the main victims, especially the worrying, overconscientious types who drive themselves too hard; also those who worry inwardly but always keep themselves under control. Four out of five of these patients are men.

To seek escape from tension in the conventional drink or cocktail usually only intensifies the damaging effects of the stress caused by tension. The effects of several glasses of strong alcohol poured on to the sensitive lining of an empty stomach before lunch or dinner are far worse than over-eating and taking meals that are too rich. Neither can the most sensible meal in the world undo the damage done by the alcohol that preceded it.

The effect of tranquilizing pills is about the same. Two hundred million dollars are spent annually on tranquilizers in the United States. The tranquilizer has a superficial effect in that it will relieve nervous or emotional tension temporarily, but when it comes to the genuine relief of physical stress conditions caused by the tension, this effect is not only illusory but a downright lie.

As we have seen, physical stress comes from the hormonal imbalance caused by disturbed glandular function. The body is maintained in equilibrium by its own chemistry, the chemistry of its glands in their hormone production. Even when we try to rectify imbalance by the administration of synthetic hormones, the result is at least dubious, possibly dangerous. What, therefore, can we expect from the administration of utterly foreign chemical substances introduced into the system to mask the signs of internal stress? All they do is give the overworked glands an additional burden to carry.

Another alleged tranquilizer is the cigarette. The American Cancer Society has published results of a survey carried out on smoking involving 200,000 persons. These results have nothing to do with cancer, but a great deal to do with physical stress. (This could mean that one of these days cancer may be added to the lengthening list of stress diseases.)

Dr. Paul Gofman of the University of California found that cigarette smoking is associated with an increase in certain fatty (cholesterol) substances in the blood related to coronary arterial hardening, and thus to heart attack risk.

A cigarette smoker, says Dr. Gofman, raises his blood pressure by 20 percent while smoking two cigarettes consecutively. Anyone who gets through two packs of cigarettes a day raises his blood pressure on average six percent above that of a nonsmoker. Regular smokers, he found, had from one-and-a-half to twice as many heart attacks as a non-cigarette smoker.

There are also the people who seek release from tension —generally quite unconsciously—not in alcohol, tobacco or tranquilizing drugs but in stuffing themselves with food. They are not popular with life insurance companies; their death rate, for instance, when they are twenty percent or more overweight, is one-third higher than that of people insured as standard risks. And, in fact, people who are 15 to 20 lbs. *under* average weight are found to live longest. This raises the question: are the thin also healthier than average and overweights?

The researches of Dr. McCay of Cornell University throw some light on this matter. He found that the diseases of old age are delayed in animals if they are kept thin. Another researcher, Paul Ehrich, the German bacteriologist, found it impossible to transplant tumors into partially starved mice.

There are, of course, the obese who eat sparingly: but in such cases obesity is nearly always a sign of glandular imbalance, and therefore a physical stress. Some of the automatic biological functions have been disturbed—not perhaps last week or last year but as far back as puberty or childhood. And their internal physical stress may also have current emotional tensions to aggravate it. There are indeed people who worry themselves fat. On the surface seemingly calm, they are always secretly brooding. It is their hormonal imbalance which has primarily produced obesity.

Finally there are the people who are suffering from total stress—those whose adaption mechanism has already broken down. Almost invariably such patients are advised by their doctors simply to rest. Enforced inactivity in such circumstances may be actually harmful in that it will cause more stress than normal or slightly reduced activity.

Psychological treatment can, however, be helpful in cases of psychosomatic illness, and some of the modern "mind drugs" may bring superficial relief to the somato-psychic cases. But whatever the treatment given, it usually takes a long time for the patient to recover and find his physical and mental balance. The physical damage resulting from years of stress is not easily reached and cured by psychological methods or mind drugs.

But these cases respond very well indeed to the biological approach. Cell therapists see more of "manager diseases," "executive collapse" and other versions of the stress syndrome than almost any other type of illness. These cases are among the most satisfactory to treat. Even when everything in the poor old body is dysfunctioning in protest against years of abuse, it usually recovers quite spectacularly after cell injections, proving that the human system really is tough after all.

Such results come from working with and not against Nature. Instead of doing violence to the natural processes of the body—suppressing, stimulating, taking over impaired function and imitating it in a crude, makeshift manner by means of drugs—the injected materials, the vital young cells, provide emergency food which is absorbed readily where it is needed. These living units of energy set up a chain reaction of cell reproduction where the worn-out or diseased human cells are no longer capable of splitting and multiplying for themselves, and the tired, used-up tissue is gently rebuilt, revitalized and restored to normal function by the biologically regenerative process which starts with the cell.

14

The British Practice

I<small>T</small> was in 1953 that Dr. Ernest Stephan first brought cell therapy to London.

Although he had been born in Holland and brought up there, he was in fact of Anglo-French parentage and held both nationalities. In the variety of his educational background and intellectual interests he was a somewhat similar type of man to the famous Swiss doctor whose work he was to discover and introduce to this country.

Having taken a medical degree at Leiden University, he went on to Zurich, where he studied under Jung and became a Doctor of Philosophy. After that came the school of Homeopathy in Berlin, and he was still there when the Second World War broke out.

He was arrested by the Germans and passed the war years in internment camps in Europe, being eventually released from a camp in Poland in 1945 by the Russians.

The practice he opened two years later in London, together with a sister practice in Munich, was devoted in those early days to nerve manipulation, a method of physical treatment he had learned from an Indian teacher while studying homeopathy in Berlin, a treatment incidentally which we still carry on today side by side with the cell therapy practice.

The Niehans' method of cellular therapy first came to my father's notice in Munich, where he saw it being used in hospitals in the treatment of Mongol children. The results obtained so impressed him that he went to see Paul Niehans in Switzerland and made arrangements to study the therapy fully.

He had in mind then not to replace the nerve manipulation given in his clinics with cell therapy, but just to use this new and controversial treatment on selected patients who were not responding well to the manipulative massage.

To begin with he gave only very small doses of cells but the results were so outstanding that word got around, and more and more patients arrived at his consulting rooms asking for the treatment—so that, almost in spite of himself, his cell therapy practice grew and inevitably attracted publicity.

The sensational "eternal youth" angle of the theory made popular newspaper headlines and my father came in for a good deal of criticism. He was called a "quack" and a "rogue" and was finally brought to court to defend his right to call himself a doctor of medicine at all.

For certain family reasons he was unwilling to give proof of his bona fides in open court, but in a private interview with the judge presiding over the case, he convinced the latter of the authenticity of his qualifications. The judge returned to the courtroom, expressed himself satisfied that the man, if not the name, was all he claimed to be, and dismisssed the case.

The cell therapy practice continued to grow. But my father's wartime experiences were catching up with him: he was a very sick man. And ironically his illness—a virus infection contracted during his years of imprisonment—was of a kind which made treatment by the therapy he was using to cure others useless to him. A virus infection is one of the contradictions to cell therapy, and must be cleared up before the injections can be effective.

It was because he knew that he could not be sure of many more years, that, in spite of the fact that I was only 15 at the time and still at school, my father began teaching me the rudiments of the practice. His intention then was that I should continue to study with the idea of going to university to take my medical degree, as he had done, but, at the same time, that I should try to learn everything he could teach me about, first, nerve manipulation, and then the practice of and application of cell therapy.

There is no doubt I learned fast. Perhaps, and this is what I myself believe, it was simply that my father was a superb teacher. But whatever the reason, perhaps almost without knowing it, I realized that time was short. By early 1961, while still in my teens, I had my own patients for nerve manipulation, treating them in the evenings and on the occasional afternoon when I had no lessons. Gradually, too, I began to take a more active part in the cell therapy practice. I studied the subject closely with my father, at first just assisting him in the application of the treatments, later coming in on the consultations with patients and finally, in the last months before his death in 1965, helping him in the preparation of treatments.

It was, however, when I learned that my father had at most six months to live that I had to make an important decision; I had to choose either to continue with my medical studies, or to forget these and devote all my time to studying cell therapy and to learning everything I could from a man whom I—and not only I but many others—believed to be a great man.

After careful thought I chose the second course. I decided that all the work which had been put into this practice could not stop and finish with the death of my father. It would have been too long a gap if I had continued with my medical studies, qualified as a doctor, and then come back to it, and I was determined that these were the fields I should continue to work in. The success of the practice since my father's death has proved that I made the right choice. But there has never been any doubt in my mind about how much I owe not only to my father, who worked on, teaching and guiding me until literally a few days before he died, but also to those of his friends and colleagues on the Continent with whom he had always collaborated closely in his cell therapy work. In those early days of trying to carry on alone immediately after my father's death, their help and encouragement were something I can never repay or forget. I should like to specially thank Professor Paul Niehans, the originator of cell therapy, for his personal help and assistance during our many meetings.

Dr. A. Griffel of Zurich, consultant to Pharmacon, the firm which prepared the cells used in treatment, went on giving me his time and he took endless pains in teaching me the finer points of the therapy and seeing that I was always kept up to date with all the latest developments as they took place.

Dr. W. Michel, head of the Niehans clinic in Switzerland, himself showed me the dissection and preparation of live cells for treatment.

The late Professor H. Dykerhoff, creator of the cell extract preparation Regeneressen used instead of the whole cell preparation in cases of great age or physical weakness, continued to carry out the Abderhalden tests for me as he had for my father, and to give me help and advice in the complexities of diagnosis; as today does Professor Dykerhoff's successor, Professor H. Gaus.

Dr. J. Stein of Heidelberg, too, who is at present in charge of the preparation and production of cells, has always given me invaluable assistance.

And the more the practice has grown, the greater has always become my enthusiasm for and belief in this work. It is my considered view that Professor Niehans is a truly great man who has been criticized and accused by people without knowledge. And the proof of this lies in the fact that not only has cell therapy remained for nearly forty years, but the list of people who have undergone it is so impressive it cannot be ignored.

Great statesmen, famous actors, international millionaires who have at their finger tips the best medical advice available in the world still have cell therapy. Why? Because it works.

Those who criticize and condemn should first try to understand its principles and its limitations.

It is not the universal panacea for all ills—of course it isn't; and no one who knows anything about it has ever suggested that it was. Cell therapy is a scientific logical treatment based on research and the development of biological repair.

It is not, in fact, very far removed from organ transplants but, because it is different, it is called "wrong." Yet its successes cannot be disputed, its results cannot be disregarded and its effects are so obvious that they demand, deserve and get a second look.

The British practice is growing all the time, and people who come to ask for cell treatment today are not just the rich wanting to be young again, they are people who are tired, jaded, nervous, anxious, unhappy or downright ill, people who feel that they are just not getting what they should from life and who have found no answer to their health problems in the pills and tablets of orthodox medicine.

They have heard about cell therapy and what it might be able to do for them. They come interested and hopeful. And they are seldom disappointed.

These are not just claims made in the air. The case histories of close on 2,000 people who have had cell treatment at the British Cell Therapy Centre since it opened its rooms 23 years ago provide powerful and indisputable support for them.

The following pages give just a small selection of typical cases.

The patients concerned have allowed the discussion of their cases provided their names are not mentioned, and also, with the same proviso, the publication of relevant parts of their letters. These patients are therefore identified by their number of the Abderhalden test result reports.

Case History No. 62190:
Patient: Male
Age: 64 years

Occupation: Retired army officer
Date of first consultation: February 14th, 1962
Pulse rate 80; blood pressure 138/74 (both normal)
Patient complained of: T.B. at the age of 8, from which he had fully recovered. He was gassed in the First World War and had oxygen cure; now suffers from bronchitis. He had prostate inflammation and had mercury cure. Now suffers from duodenal ulcers and urticaria, and from cramps in hands, legs and face. He is gradually becoming impotent; has inflammation of the joints and bad circulation. Also suffers from emphysema and is always short of breath. His nails are brittle, his skin is dry and he has headaches.

Abderhalden test result showed dysfunction of: Frontal Lobe, Temporal Lobe, Cerebellum, Thalamus, Kidney, Liver, Spleen, Heart, Arteries, Stomach, Parathyroid, Thyroid, Hypothalamus, Pancreas, Suprarenal Prostate, Testes.

His cramps would be caused by the parathyroid gland; the Spleen and Hypothalamus would account for his cold feeling; Heart and Arteries would account for his shortness of breath.

Injections of the following were given: Testes, Placenta, Hypothalamus, Thalamus, Suprarenal Cortex, Liver, Parathyroid, Heart, Arteries, Spleen, Cerebellum, Stomach— a total of twelve injections in three sessions with three days rest between each one.

The patient reported he was much better, he was able to do more and was much less tired, the cramps went away, he did not feel the cold so much and he improved sexually.

The patient wrote in a letter:

"In March, 1962, when I was sixty-four years old, I was in poor health, chronically exhausted, very breathless after slight exertion, normal pulse rate 95, subject to acute cramps and compelled to take the equivalent of 25 mg hydrocortisone daily for adrenal insufficiency. The Abderhalden tests confirmed poor heart condition, considerable atrophy of the suprarenal glands and parathyroid glands and a lowered efficiency of liver and kidneys.

I received 22 units of cell injections including, among others, placenta, heart, arteries, parathyroid gland, suprarenal cortex and gonad. After about six weeks I noticed a very definite and considerable increase in health. My heart was stronger, I was no longer as weak and breathless, my pulse rate dropped to 70½, I stopped having cramps and I was able to manage on one quarter of my maintenance dose of cortisone. The results were so good that in March 1963 I had further cell treatment. The results were less spectacular but gave further improvement in general health. In 1969 at the age of 71, I am considering further cell treatment. . . ."

Case History No. 144404
Patient: Male
Age: 60
Occupation: Surveyor
Date of first Consultation: June 2nd, 1967

The patient complained of lack of energy; he was an enthusiastic tennis player and wanted to continue to be able to play. His memory was not as good as it could be, and he used to forget names which was bad for his work. He also felt tense and had some difficulty passing water.

Pulse rate: 100 (too high); blod pressure: 140/90 (acceptable).

Abderhalden test result showed dysfunction of Frontal Lobe, Cerebellum, Thalamus, and Hypothalamus, as well as Kidney, Liver, Spleen, Heart, Arteries, Bone Marrow, Thyroid, Pituitary Anterior Lobe, Pancreas and Suprarenal gland.

The lack of energy would be associated with the Suprarenal glands; his memory troubles with the Frontal Lobe and Hypothalamus, which would also be involved in his feelings of tension.

Injections of the following cells were given: Placenta, Testes, Hypothalamus, Liver, Suprarenal gland—a total of six injections in one session with three days rest following.

In August 1967 the patient reported that he was feeling better, he was much more relaxed. He felt better able to organize his business life and his memory and concentration had greatly improved. His previous difficulty in passing water had cleared completely. He wrote in a letter:

"Dear Mr. Stephan, I have no reason whatever for wishing to conceal the fact that in my experience your treatment has been of real benefit particularly from the viewpoint of a professional person in that it has enabled me to give my work far greater energy and concentration than previously and to carry an almost unbearable load of work without breaking down either physically or mentally despite the fact that I have been continuously, during the past three months, in homes with colds and influenza and have been getting around in the worst possible weather, often getting wet and chilled to the marrow but without any untoward effect. The hours of work have been greatly extended for me during this period and I have had to work most evenings up to midnight and very often at 5:30 in the morning as well, and during the day have been motoring all the time, so that I could get no rest. Despite all this, my blood pressure recently taken was 140/80 and my heart pronounced to be entirely normal, and as one would expect a much younger man's to be. I am sure it would therefore help anyone who may be called upon to withstand any sort of 'endurance test.' With kind regards. . . ."

Case History No. 117924
Patient: Female
Age: 53 years
Profession: Principal of private school
Date of first consultation: May 11th, 1966

The patient complained of mental tiredness, lack of energy and intermittent pains all over her body, especially in her neck, which were causing her great discomfort. Her memory and concentration were not good, and she put weight on very easily. She also felt the cold badly and her skin was very dry.

Pulse rate: 56 (too low); blood pressure: 150/90 (acceptable).

Abderhalden test result showed dysfunction of Frontal Lobe, Cerebellum, Thalamus, Hypothalamus, Kidney, Liver, Spleen, Heart, Bone Marrow, Thyroid, Pituitary Anterior Lobe and Suprarenal gland.

The Thyroid would account for her weight problem and this, together with the Suprarenal glands, would account for her dry skin and lack of energy. The Suprarenal gland would also account for the intermittent pains throughout her body. The fact that she felt the cold would be due to the Spleen and Bone Marrow dysfunction, and also to some degree to the Thyroid.

Injections of the following cells were given: Placenta, Ovary, Liver, Spleen, Thyroid, Suprarenal gland—a total of six injections given in one session with three days rest in bed following.

In September 1966 the patient reported that she felt very much better, she had much more energy, and was looking better. Her aches and pains had diminished and her memory and concentration had greatly improved.

The patient wrote in a letter:

"Dear Mr. Stephan, I am writing to tell you that after the injections there was a decided improvement of concentration and a general feeling of well-being. The rheumatic pains lessened enormously and feelings of depression disappeared. I am sleeping better and I must say I have a much more optimistic outlook.

"When I came to you I was very tired and jaded but now I have my old energy back. There are many intangible things that have improved, but altogether life is much more enjoyable. Thank you. Yours sincerely, . . ."

Case History No. 435191
Patient: Female
Age: 5 years
Date of first consultation: September 3rd, 1966

The patient is mongol.

Treatment, given in three sessions, was as follows:

1st treatment: Cerebellum, Pituitary, Frontal Lobe, Thalamus, Thyroid—a total of five injections given in one session with three days rest in bed following.

2nd treatment: Cerebellum, Pituitary, Frontal Lobe, Thymus, Thyroid—given again in one session with three days rest in bed following.

[147]

3rd treatment: Thymus, Thyroid, Hypothalamus, Pituitary, Frontal Lobe—again with three days rest in bed.

The mother reported that the child walked a lot better and that her facial expression had improved. She had gained seven pounds and her intelligence had improved. The mother also felt that her eyesight was better and that she seemed much more interested.

When the child had to return for the second treatment, she had to be seen in a different room because she remembered the room and the treatment. The final treatment had to be given at home because she did not like coming to London since she linked her visits with the treatments.

On December 12th, 1966 her mother wrote in a letter (personal parts of this letter are omitted for obvious reasons):

". . . my husband is happy with the improvement in Elia and wishes to carry on with the treatment . . . Elia is going along well but misses terribly her daily walk to the park. She is constantly asking me to go to the park. . . . You will probably be interested to know that Elia can now turn a skipping rope very well with the correct rhythm, so at least she can now join in a game of skipping with the other children. Of course she skips in her own little way—more of a jump than a skip—but perhaps this will improve with time. Her memory, too, is definitely improving. . . ."

Case History No. 59673
Patient: Female
Age: 41 years
Occupation: Secretary-Personal Assistant
Date of first consultation: July 18th, 1962

The patient complained of feeling unwell for some time; she suffered from pains over all her body, and from very bad headaches and constriction of her throat. She felt very tense, particularly at the time of her period, and had been having psychiatric treatment for some time. She suffered from extreme temperature changes in her hands and feet, and from sudden bursts of perspiration and palpitations. She slept very badly and woke up feeling awful in the mornings.

Pulse rate: 80 (normal); blood pressure: 108/62 (too low).

Abderhalden test result showed dysfunction of Cerebellum, Thalamus, Hypothalamus, Heart, Kidney, Liver, Spleen, Arteries, Bone Marrow, Thyroid, Pituitary Anterior Lobe, Suprarenal glands, Ovary.

The Hypothalamus dysfunction would account for her temperature change and pains. The Parathyroid would affect the palpitations and constriction of the throat. The Spleen and Suprarenal gland would account for her general debility.

Injections were given of Placenta, Ovary, Cerebellum, Spleen, Suprarenal Cortex, Parathyroid and Hypothalamus —a total of seven injections in one session with three days rest in bed.

The patient wrote in a letter dated October 2nd, 1963

". . . I came to your consulting rooms . . . I realize now in a far worse state of health than I myself knew at the time! I should like you to know, in fact I should like the whole world to know, how very different and well I feel in comparison with many years previously. I came to accept these as common to many people . . . and persuaded there just was no cure. Today I know differently and experience the comfort of reasonably good health, together with a sense of well-being and the all important peace of mind for which I cannot be thankful enough to God and your work. . . . Once again may I congratulate you on your amazing cure which, I must add, has withstood quite a considerable test over the past months . . . best wishes for your continued success. . . ."

Case History No. 147922
Patient: Male
Age: 65 years
Occupation: Retired company director
Date of first consultation: May 13th, 1966
    The patient complained of lack of energy and difficulty in concentrating. Had woken up one morning without feeling in arms and legs. Suffered from cramps in his legs in bed and found himself very sensitive to temperature changes. His sex life had been unsatisfactory for many years and he put on weight easily.
    Pulse rate: 75; blood pressure 160/90 (both acceptable).
    Abderhalden test result showed dysfunction of—Frontal Lobe, Cerebellum, Thalamus, Hypothalamus, Kidney, Liver, Spleen, Heart, Arteries, Bone Marrow, Thyroid, Pituitary Anterior Lobe, Pancreas, Suprarenal gland. Injections of the following cell preparations were given: Placenta, Testes, Liver, Spleen, Heart, Pancreas and Suprarenal gland—a total of seven injections administered in one session with three days rest in bed following.
    In September 1966 the patient reported he was feeling better, that his previous pains had gone and that his sex life had improved. He did not feel the cold so intensely

and he was able to play much more golf, and also concentrate better.

He wrote in a letter:

"When I had the cellular injections I had them with an open mind and did not tell anybody.

"Years before I had fallen heavily on my shoulder and frequently had pains. After the injections they were worse than ever and then completely disappeared and have never returned.

"There were other manifestations such as almost painful discharge at the corner of my eyes which cleared up and have never reappeared. I also remember slight pains in my head, I have never had headaches, and these pains soon went away and have never come back.

"I was most interested to see if people would remark on my health and soon one of my golf cronies was pestering me to know why my golf was so much better. Other people were saying that I was far more sociable and were wondering why. Kindest regards, . . ."

Case History No. 49174
Patient: Female
Age: 54 years
Profession: Concert Pianist
First consultation: August 22nd, 1960

Patient complained of a feeling of growing exhaustion for the past 18 months. She slept too long, but woke feeling still tired. Her concentration and memory were very poor, and she felt unable to carry on with her music because her fingers were too tired. Her skin was in a poor condition and morally she was very low.

Pulse rate: 96 (a little fast); blood pressure 104/68 (too low).

Abderhalden test result showed dysfunction of Thalamus, Hypothalamus, Frontal Lobe, Kidney, Liver, Heart, Spleen, Thyroid and Suprarenal gland. Injections of the following cell preparations were given: Placenta, Ovary, Hypothalamus, Thalamus, Thyroid, Liver, Spleen, Frontal Lobe, Suprarenal Cortex, Kidney and Heart—a total of eleven injections, administered in two sessions with three days rest in bed between each session.

In July 1961 the patient reported she was feeling much better; she was also looking better.

In 1962 the patient had a second smaller treatment following another Abderhalden test.

This time the treatment given used the following cell preparations: Placenta, Hypothalamus, Cerebellum, Suprarenal Cortex, Suprarenal gland and Thalamus, also Ovary cells: a total of six injections given this time in one session, followed by three days rest in bed.

Shortly after the treatment the patient reported feeling once again very much better and that her health generally had greatly improved.

The patient had further treatments in 1965 and 1968, and continues to report good health.

She wrote in a letter:

"Dear Mr. Stephan, I would call cell treatment the miracle of the age.

"When I went to see your father I was so exhausted and physically depleted that the laboratory test showed me to be an old 65. I was in fact only 45.

"I had the first treatment and my whole life began to change in a matter of weeks. It happened just as your father said it would—that one lived one's life in retrospect feeling and remembering back 5, 10 and 15 years. I have had several treatments since then, the recent ones with you since your father died. I remember so vividly the day I went to see him, first knowing nothing about him or the treatment except what I had read and yet having talked to him, I trusted him absolutely, knowing myself to be in the presence of an exceptional and truly great man.

"The whole success and development of my life has been made possible by the cell treatment and the great skill and knowledge with which you and your father applied it.

"I live an 18-hour day to the full and have health, vitality and looks that reflect both. You have achieved this for me and no one could be more grateful than I. I could never thank you enough.

"That cell treatment is not generally accepted and practiced here is to me a crime against humanity. Yours sincerely, . . ."

Case History No. 80831
Patient: Male
Age: 79 years
Occupation: Retired Q.C.
Date of first consultation: November 24th, 1964
Pulse rate 78 (normal); blood pressure 122/62 (a bit low).

The patient complained of cystitis, constipation, allergy, continued tonsil infections and feeling lethargic all the time. His memory and concentration were failing. He suffered from lumbago attacks and palpitations. He felt nervous, tense and highly strung.

The Abderhalden test result showed dysfunction of: Frontal Lobe, Cerebellum, Thalamus, Hypothalamus, Kidney, Liver, Spleen, Heart, Arteries, Stomach, Gall bladder, Bladder, Bone Marrow, Thyroid, Pancreas, Suprarenal gland.

The Frontal Lobe, Cerebellum, Hypothalamus and Thalamus would account for the tense feeling and failing memory and concentration: the Bone Marrow, Spleen and Suprarenal glands together with the Thyroid would account for the lethargic feeling and palpitations.

Injections of the following were given: Placenta, Testes, Frontal Lobe, Cerebellum, Thalamus, Kidney, Liver, Spleen, Heart, Stomach, Bone Marrow, Thyroid, Pancreas and Suprarenal gland—a total of fourteen injections in two sessions with three days rest between each.

The patient wrote in a letter:

"When I decided to try cellular therapy in 1964, my health was in an unsatisfactory state. I was suffering from cystitis and exhaustion and had no energy. My symptoms as I detailed them at the time were—exhaustion, a tendency toward constipation, backache, cold hands and feet, palpitations and I was nervous.

"After receiving some 8 injections I spent 2-3 days in bed on advice, though I felt no inconvenience beyond a slight stiffness in the back. During the next five years there has been a gradual amelioration and today when I am in my 84th year I am able to walk and take vigorous exercise without inconvenience.

"The improvement has been so gradual that it is difficult to point to anything definite but I can say after 5 years during which I should have shown signs of increasing old age, I feel I am to all intents younger than in 1964."

[154]

Case History No. 125932
Patient: Male
Age: 74 years
Occupation: Retired managing director
Date of first consultation: June 7th, 1966
Pulse rate: 60 (low); blood pressure 150/60 (normal)

The patient complained of intermittent claudication (caused by arterial spasms), strain of heart, difficulty in walking, constipation. His memory and concentration were failing. He was overweight. His skin, nails and hair were in low condition. He felt congestion in his chest.

The Abderhalden test result showed dysfunction of Frontal Lobe, Cerebellum, Thalamus, Hypothalamus, Spondylus, Cartilago, Synovia, Kidney, Liver, Spleen, Heart, Arteries, Stomach, Gall Bladder, Bone Marrow, Lungs, Parathyroid, Thyroid, Pancreas, Suprarenal gland.

Injections of the following cells were given: Placenta, Testes, Kidney, Liver, Heart, Spleen, Thyroid—a total of seven injections in one session with three days rest following.

The patient wrote in a letter:

"It was nice to receive your letter enquiring how I was keeping these days, I found it waiting on my return from a four-week cruise around the Mediterranean. It's astonishing to think that over seven years ago at the age of 70 when (on my doctor's advice) I first received your cell treatment I could then hardly walk 100 yards without intense pain in my legs. This was of course due to hardened arteries and intermittent claudication, and now after receiving your cell treatment four times over the past seven years I walk a mile without the discomfort and exhaustion I felt seven years ago. All my friends tell me that I look

[155]

much younger these days and I certainly feel it. The aging process seems to have reversed itself in my case over the past seven years. This, I am sure, is due only to the help I have received from your treatment.

"I was being massaged at a local hydro a little while ago when the masseur remarked that my skin (which as you know used to be very dry and hard) looked more like a person's in his early 50's rather than one in his late 70's.

"I am looking forward to seeing you again at the end of this year when I hope to receive your cell treatment for the 5th time. . . ."

Case History No. 98115
Patient: Male
Age: 33
Occupation: Company Director
Date of first consultation: August 10th, 1965

Patient complained of extreme tension which had been getting steadily worse. He was taking daily 16×½-gr. Sodium Amytal (tranquilizer) and 12×Librium (antidepressant). He had suffered from acute depression ever since 1958, and from headaches which travelled from the base of the spine over the top of the head. Although he slept well, he always woke up feeling awful. He felt incapable of meeting people, and his memory and concentration were bad. He had difficulty holding water. He had no sex life and he tired very easily. He used to lose the feeling in his hands and he felt the cold a great deal. The hormone treatment prescribed by his doctors in the past had put up his weight to 224 pounds. He wanted to stop taking the tablets.

Pulse rate: 80 (normal); blood pressure 118/60 (a little low).

Abderhalden test results showed dysfunction in the Frontal Lobe, Diencephalon, Cerebellum, Hypothalamus, Thalamus, Kidney, Liver, Spleen, Heart, Arteries, Muscle, Stomach, Bone Marrow, Thyroid, Pituitary Anterior Lobe, Pancreas, Suprarenal gland, Testes.

Dysfunction of the Frontal Lobe, Diencephalon, Thalamus and Hypothalamus would account for his depression and mental difficulties, the Hypothalamus for his pains, the Pituitary Anterior Lobe for his sexual difficulties, and the Suprarenal glands for his lack of energy.

Injections of the following were given: Placenta, Testes, Frontal Lobe, Cerebellum, Stammganglien, Hypothalamus, Liver, Spleen, Muscles, Pituitary Anterior Lobe, Suprarenal gland, Testes—a total of twelve injections in two sessions with three days in bed following each session.

In December 1965 the patient reported he was feeling better, the pains in the spine and head had gone. He felt much more confident and the loss of feeling in his hands had disappeared. He felt much more refreshed in the mornings and his sex life had improved. He did not feel the cold so much.

The patient wrote in a letter:

"Dear Mr. Stephan, In giving this final of a series of oral reports to you following my cell treatment of last October I feel I must stress my deep gratitude to you for the benefits I have enjoyed from the treatment, and for your advice, interest and help given during my visits since. At this time I am feeling better in health than at any time within my memory and an uplift in confidence which enables me to go about my daily work with zest and enjoyment.

[157]

"All this change seems to me to be an incredible thing when I look back on so many years of poor health and the feeling of hopelessness that went with it as I visited hospitals, doctors, psychiatrists and Harley Street specialists to no avail. Apart from trying to digest a tremendous amount of advice, virtually the only treatment I received was in the form of tablets, this as time went on building up to an intake of 30 each day, comprising 16 Amytal and the balance in equal doses of Librium and Marsalid.

"On my first visit to you I was impressed by what you had to say and in your confidence that you could treat me successfully. Perhaps your insistence against the use of drugs was a big incentive to me for while I realized the difficulty of giving these up, I really felt a hopelessness about my benefits from them.

"I astounded myself and, I believe, many others in giving up these tablets in a short period of time, as you insisted that this was necessary before having the cell treatment.

"Now after about four months following this treatment I am enjoying wonderfully good health with a build up of confidence which goes with it. Not once have I taken any of these past drugs and not once have I had a desire to do so. I cannot express adequately my gratitude to you and to the cell treatment for the change made to my life and hopes for the future. As you suggest I shall keep in touch with you and report on progress. Sincerely yours, . . ."

Epilogue

On September 1, 1971, just as this book was going to press, news came that Dr. Niehans had passed away in his sleep at his clinic at Montreux at the age of 89. He had been active up to the time of his death and had just recently performed one of his more than 50,000 operations, a record equaled by very few surgeons.